America's Most Successful Cardiovascular Health Program

The Vitamin Program That
Conquers the Hearts of America

Matthias Rath, M.D.

Published and distributed by Health Now
387 Ivy Street, San Francisco, CA 94102 U.S.A.
To order call 1-800-624-2442.

ISBN 0-9638768-2-1

To Melvin Belli

For His 88th Birthday

Table of Contents

	Page
Invitation to my Readers	8
10 Step Program to Optimum Cardiovascular Health	12
A Daily Program of Essential Nutrients for Optimum Cardiovascular Health	14
Cellular Medicine - the New Understanding of Health and Disease	15
Cellular Medicine	16
The Principles of Cellular Medicine	17
Essential Nutrients - Biological Fuel for Millions of Cells	18
Cellular Medicine and Cardiovascular Disease	20
Cellular Medicine - Breakthrough for	
Coronary Heart Disease Patients	25
Arrhythmia Patients	65
Heart Failure Patients	91
High Blood Pressure Patients	111
Diabetic Patients	123
Prevention of Cardiovascular Disease	133
Other Encouraging Letters	147
America's Most Successful Cardiovascular Health Program - Compared to Other Approaches: Biological Targets - Biological Versatility - Safety	151
Milestones of Cellular Medicine	156
Acknowledgments	158
References	159

Dear Reader:

Only a few times in human history medical breakthroughs are made that lead to the control of worldwide epidemics and improve the lives of hundreds of millions of people. Over the recent years I have led a scientific breakthrough leading to the control of the cardiovascular epidemic. This book is the first comprehensive documentation that the battle against cardiovascular diseases can be won for this generation and for all future generations of mankind.

Until today, heart attacks and strokes kill every second person in America. Moreover, tens of millions of Americans have already been diagnosed with one or more of the following cardiovascular conditions:

- High Blood Pressure   50 Million Americans
- Arrhythmia   8   Million Americans
- Coronary Heart Disease   6   Million Americans
- Stroke   3   Million Americans

According to the World Health Organization, over one billion people living today will die from cardiovascular disease world-wide, if this epidemic cannot be controlled.

Fortunately, we now have the opportunity to control the cardiovascular epidemic. Heart attacks, strokes and many other cardiovascular conditions are primarily caused by long-term deficiencies in vitamins and other essential nutrients. This medical advance is documented in my two books *"Eradicating Heart Disease"* and *"Why Animals Don't Get Heart Attacks"*. In these books I also presented my "Ten Step Program to Optimum Cardiovascular Health", comprising a daily intake of vitamins and other essential nutrients in combination with a healthy life style. By now, over 20,000 Americans follow this program on a daily basis for preventive purposes and as an adjunct to conventional therapy.

America's Most Successful Cardiovascular Health Program is the first comprehensive documentation of the health benefits of this natural cardiovascular program. It is entirely composed of letters from grateful patients who have greatly benefited from this program. The results are so encouraging that many people have written to us about the health improvements when they started this program. We decided to compile these letters and make them available to all those who are interested to improve their cardiovascular health naturally.

'America's Most Successful Cardiovascular Health Program' is an invaluable documentation

- *For millions of heart patients* who will find valuable information how to improve their health naturally. Thousands of patients with angina pectoris, high blood pressure, arrhythmia, heart failure, diabetes, high cholesterol levels and other health conditions are following my cardiovascular health program. They report about significant health improvements - beyond anything achieved with drugs alone or with life style changes only. As a patient I recommend that you to start this program as soon as possible. Inform your doctor about this program by taking this book with you. Document your health improvements and share them with your doctor. Do not stop your prescription medication without consulting with your doctor. The natural cardiovascular health program in this book is an adjunct to conventional therapy - not a substitute for your doctor's advice.

- *For hundreds of millions of people from teen age to the silver generation.* The natural cardiovascular health program in this book is primarily an easy to follow daily program for all those among my readers who want to prevent cardiovascular conditions in the first place. Deficiencies in vitamins and other essential nutrients are a frequent cause of different cardiovascular conditions. Optimum daily intake of the right essential nutrients in combination with a healthy life style is the best way to enjoy a long and healthy life.

- *For doctors and other health professionals.* For the first time a natural cardiovascular health program is available that is scientifically based and therefore can deliver reproducible health benefits in patients. This natural health program is already a valuable option for many medical professionals as a basic health program for patients. The medical breakthrough in different cardiovascular areas at the same time is based on our new understanding of Cellular Medicine. The scientific basis of Cellular Medicine and its impact on a variety of cardiovascular conditions is documented throughout this book.

'America's Most Successful Cardiovascular Health Program' should be a "must read"

- **For every health insurance company, health maintenance organization, and other health care providers in America.** Consider recommending this effective, safe and natural cardiovascular program as a basic health care measure to your clients and patients. The cost/benefit ratio of a large scale implementation of this program will allow you to offer very competitive premiums while maintaining and improving the standard of health care.

- **For the President of the United States, the members of US Congress and other political decision takers.** According to this year's Economic Report of the President to the Congress, aggregate health care costs in the United States are currently running at fourteen percent of the gross domestic product, equaling more than four trillion (four thousand billion) US dollars. Expenses for the cardiovascular epidemic are the single largest portion of this astronomic sum. Government, corporations and millions of Americans each carry about one third of this huge economic burden. America's Most Successful Cardiovascular Health Program is a public health program and a decisive answer to the escalating health care crisis. Systematic implementation of this preventive health care program as a public health measure could save billions of dollars for the federal and state governments as well as for thousands of communities across America.

- **For corporate America.** Every corporation, large and small, should have a close look at this cardiovascular health program. Consider recommending this effective, safe and affordable basic health care program to all your employees. You will decisively lower the health care expenses of your company and increase your economic competitiveness nationally and internationally.

- **For millions of American people.** Skyrocketing health care costs have a profound economic impact on every American. This year's Economic Report of the President highlights that inflating health care costs were the primary reason why the average real take-home pay for millions of Americans has barely increased over the past thirty years. Therefore, every American also has a direct economic interest in the immediate and nationwide implementation of an effective, safe and affordable health care program. The sooner this basic health program is used in every doctor's office and hospital , the more money millions of Americans will save. Your savings will be substantial and will come from three areas: You will have less expenses for health care, you will have lower health insurance premiums, and you will eventually pay less taxes. Obvious health benefits and economic advantages are the reasons this cardiovascular health program is taking the hearts of millions of Americans by storm.

America's Most Successful Cardiovascular Health Program also promotes regular physical activity and a healthy diet. I recommend you to get as many essential nutrients as possible through a diet rich in vitamins, minerals and fiber. To that effect, this book also highlights nutritional information on particularly healthy foods.

In the documented letters passages containing the most important information for my readers were underlined. Everyone can read through this book with ease and understand its significance.

This testimonial book will be an ongoing documentation. In addition to clinical studies, we will continue to document the encouraging health benefits which are currently improving the daily lives of thousands of people on this program.

Just as this book may have helped you, so could you help others in the future by sharing your health improvements while following this program. I invite you to send me a short letter and we will consider publishing it in the next edition of this book.

Finally I would like to thank all those whose contribution made this book possible.

Here's to Your health, America!

                                                    Matthias Rath, M.D.

My Ten Step Program
to Optimum Cardiovascular Health

1. **Be aware of the size and function of your cardiovascular system.** Did you know that your blood vessel pipeline system measures 60,000 miles and is the largest organ in your body? Did you do know that your heart pumps 100,000 times every day, performing the greatest amount of work of all organs? Optimizing your cardiovascular health benefits your entire body and your overall health. Optimizing your cardiovascular health adds years to your life because your body is as old as your cardiovascular system.

2. **Stabilize the walls of your blood vessels.** Blood vessel instability and lesions in your blood vessel walls are primary causes for cardiovascular disease. Vitamin C is the cement of the blood vessel walls and stabilizes them. Animals don't get heart disease because they produce enough endogenous vitamin C in their livers to protect their blood vessels. In contrast, we humans develop deposits leading to heart attacks and strokes because we cannot manufacture endogenous vitamin C and generally get too few vitamins in our diet.

3. **Reverse existing deposits in your arteries without surgery.** Cholesterol and fat particles are deposited inside the blood vessel walls by means of biological adhesives. Teflon-like agents can prevent this stickiness. The amino acids lysine and proline are nature's teflon agents. Together with vitamin C they help reverse existing deposits naturally.

4. **Relax your blood vessel walls.** Deposits and spasms of the blood vessel walls are the cause of high blood pressure. Dietary supplementation of magnesium (nature's calcium antagonist) and vitamin C relax the blood vessel walls and normalize high blood pressure. The natural amino acid arginine can be of additional value.

5. **Optimize the performance of your heart**. The heart is the motor of the cardiovascular system. Like the motor of a car, the millions of muscle cells need cell fuel for optimum performance. Nature's cell fuels include: Carnitine, coenzyme Q-10, B vitamins, many nutrients and trace elements. Dietary supplementation of these essential nutrients will optimize the pumping performance of the heart and contribute to a regular heartbeat.

6. **Protect your cardiovascular pipeline from rusting.** Biological rusting, or oxidation, damages your cardiovascular system and accelerates the aging process. Vitamin C, vitamin E, beta carotene and selenium are the most important natural antioxidants. Other important antioxidants are bioflavonoids such as pycnogenol. Dietary supplementation of these antioxidants provides important rust protection for your cardiovascular system. Above all, stop smoking, because cigarette smoke accelerates the rusting of your blood vessels.

7. **Exercise regularly.** Regular physical activity is an important element of any cardiovascular health program. Moderate and regular exercise, like walking or bicycling, is ideal and can be performed by everybody.

8. **Eat a prudent diet.** The diet of our ancestors over thousands of generations shaped our metabolism and from it we can learn what is best for our bodies today. Their diet was rich in plant nutrition and high in fiber and vitamins. A diet rich in fruits and vegetables enhances your cardiovascular health today.

9. **Find time to relax.** Physical and emotional stress are cardiovascular risk factors. Schedule hours and days to relax as you would schedule your appointments. You should also know that the production of the stress hormone adrenaline uses up your body's vitamin C supply. Long-term physical or emotional stress depletes your vitamin body pool and requires dietary vitamin supplementation.

10. **Start now.** Thickening of the blood vessel walls is not only a problem of the elderly - it starts early in life. Studies have shown that first blood vessel deposits develop before age 20. Start protecting your cardiovascular system now. The earlier you start, the more years you will add to your life.

A Daily Program of Essential Nutrients
for Optimum Cardiovascular Health

VITAMINS

Vitamin C	900	- 3,000 mg
Vitamin E (d-Alpha Tocopherol)	200	- 600 I.U.
Vitamin A (Beta-Carotene)	2,500	- 8,000 I.U.
Vitamin B-1 (Thiamine)	10	- 40 mg
Vitamin B-2 (Riboflavin)	10	- 40 mg
Vitamin B-3	65	- 200 mg
Vitamin B-5 (Pantothenate)	60	- 200 mg
Vitamin B-6 (Pyridoxine)	15	- 50 mg
Vitamin B-12 (Cyanocobalamin)	30	- 100 mcg
Vitamin D	200	- 600 I.U.
Folic Acid	130	- 400 mg
Biotin	100	- 300 mcg

MINERALS

Calcium	50	- 150 mg
Magnesium	60	- 200 mg
Potassium	30	- 90 mg
Phosphate	20	- 60 mg
Zinc	10	- 30 mg
Manganese	2	- 6 mg
Copper	500	- 2,000 mcg
Selenium	30	- 100 mcg
Chromium	15	- 50 mcg
Molybdenum	6	- 20 mcg

OTHER IMPORTANT NUTRIENTS

L-Proline	150	- 500 mg
L-Lysine	150	- 500 mg
L-Carnitine	50	- 150 mg
L-Arginine	50	- 150 mg
L-Cysteine	50	- 150 mg
Inositol	50	- 150 mg
Coenzyme Q-10	10	- 30 mg
Pycnogenol	10	- 30 mg

The first values are my minimum daily recommendations for a healthy person. People and patients with additional needs can adjust accordingly.

Cellular Medicine - Our New Understanding of Health and Disease

Cellular Medicine

The purpose of this chapter is to introduce my readers, lay person and health professional alike, to the far reaching consequences of Cellular Medicine. It is this new understanding of human health and disease that provides the scientific basis for the comprehensive and multiple health benefits documented throughout this book.

Today medicine is divided into different specialties. There is the internist, the gastroenterologist, the cardiologist, the cardiovascular surgeon and many other disciplines. As useful as this specialization is, it masks the fact that our body and its organs are built of small and very similar units, the cells. Millions of cells compose the heart, the 60,000 mile long blood vessel wall and all other organs in our body.

Cellular Medicine opens up a new era in medicine. This era is characterized by a new understanding that health and disease of our body and its organs is determined at the level of millions of cells. Optimum function of these small building blocks of life means health. In contrast, impaired function of millions of cells causes impaired organ function and disease.

The era of Cellular Medicine will lead to rapid advances in many areas of medicine and human health. Throughout this century, conventional medicine has been unable to identify the causes of most of the largest health epidemics of our time, including, coronary heart disease, high blood pressure, irregular heart beat, heart failure and many other conditions affecting the lives of millions of people.

On the basis of Cellular Medicine we now understand that the underlying cause of these conditions is frequently or even primarily an impaired function of cells. The most frequent trigger of cell malfunction is an insufficient dietary intake of vitamins and other essential cell fuel needed for a multitude of biochemical functions inside the cells.

Because the cardiovascular system is mechanically the most active organ system in our body, essential nutrients are consumed in these cardiovascular cells at a high rate. Thus the primary cause of the cardiovascular epidemic is an insufficient resupplementation of vitamins and other essential nutrients in our diet.

The Principles of Cellular Medicine

1. Health and disease are determined on the level of millions of cells which compose our body and its organs.

2. Essential nutrients are needed for thousands of biochemical reactions in each cell. Chronic deficiency of these essential nutrients is the most frequent cause of malfunction of millions of body cells and the primary cause of cardiovascular disease and other diseases.

3. Cardiovascular diseases are the most frequent diseases because cardiovascular cells consume essential nutrients at a high rate due to the mechanical stress on the heart and the blood vessel wall from the heart beat and the pulse wave.

4. Optimum dietary supplementation of essential nutrients is the key to effective prevention and treatment of cardiovascular diseases as well as other chronic health conditions.

Essential Nutrients -
Biological Fuel for Millions of Cells

The cells in our body fulfill a multitude of different functions. Gland cells produce hormones, white blood cells produce antibodies, heart muscle cells generate and conduct biological electricity for the heartbeat. The specific function of each cell is determined by the genetic software program, the genes, stored in the cell core.

Despite these different functions, it is important to understand that all cells use the same carriers of bioenergy and the same biocatalysts. Many of these essential biocatalysts and bioenergy molecules cannot be produced by the body itself and have to be supplemented in our diet on a regular basis.

Among the most important essential nutrients for the proper function of each cell in our body are vitamins, certain amino acids, minerals and trace elements. Like in a real factory, every "cell factory" needs these cell fuels to produce such biological products as hormones, antibodies or biological electricity. Without optimum intake of these essential nutrients the function of millions of cells becomes impaired, leading to impaired organ function and to the development of diseases.

The concept that diseases start at the level of cells is not new. One and a half centuries ago the German pathologist Rudolf Virchow introduced "Cellular Pathology" - the discovery that diseases are caused by cellular malfunction. Virchow's "Cellular Pathology" remains one of the cornerstones of pathology and medicine until today. While Rudolf Virchow correctly identified the most frequent causes of diseases, he could not find the most frequent remedy to cellular malfunction - vitamins and other essential nutrients were not discovered until after his death .

Even after the structural identification of most vitamins and other essential nutrients during the first half of this century, their decisive role for optimum cellular function and for optimum health was not recognized or not accepted by conventional medicine. The age of Cellular Medicine now closes this circle for the benefit of everyone living today and for all generations to come.

Essential Nutrients Catalyze
Thousands of Biochemical Reactions
in Each Cell

Important Biocatalysts:

- Vitamin B-1
- Vitamin B-2
- Vitamin B-3
- Vitamin B-5
- Vitamin B-6
- Vitamin B-12
- Vitamin C
- Carnitine
- Coenzyme Q10
- Minerals
- Trace Elements

One Single Cell Magnified

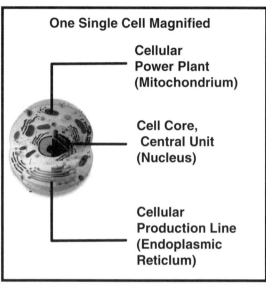

Cellular
Power Plant
(Mitochondrium)

Cell Core,
 Central Unit
(Nucleus)

Cellular
Production Line
(Endoplasmic
Reticlum)

The metabolic software program
of each cell is exactly determined
by the genetic information in
each cell core.

Essential nutrients are needed
as biocatalysts and as carriers
of bioenergy in each cell.
Both functions are essential
for optimum performance of
millions of cells.

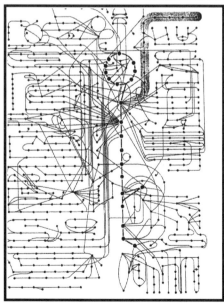

Cellular Medicine and Cardiovascular Disease

For the reasons outlined on the previous pages, the most profound impact of Cellular Medicine will be in the area of cardiovascular disease. Cardiovascular diseases, which are among the largest epidemics ever to haunt mankind, could largely be unknown in future generations.

Because of this breathtaking perspective I have summarized the close connection between Cellular Medicine and the control of cardiovascular diseases on the following pages in detail:

- The adjacent page highlights the most important cell types within the cardio-vascular system. The cells of the blood vessel wall: endothelial cells, the barrier cells between the bloodstream and the vascular wall are responsible for optimum blood viscosity; the smooth muscle cells of the vascular walls, responsible for stability and elasticity. There are the muscle cells of the heart, responsible for optimum blood pumping and for the electricity of the heartbeat. Even the corpuscles in the bloodstream are nothing other than cells, responsible for oxygen and nutrient transport, defense, wound healing and many other functions.

- The following pages summarize the consequences of long-term deficiencies in essential nutrients for the heart and the vascular system. Deficiency of essential nutrients in millions of *heart muscle cells* leads to an impaired function of the heart. The most frequent consequences are irregular heart beat (arrhythmia) and heart failure (shortness of breath, edema and fatigue).

- Deficiency of essential nutrients in millions of *vascular wall cells* impairs the function of the vascular walls. The most frequent consequences are high blood pressure and thickening of the arteries, leading to atherosclerotic deposits, heart attacks and strokes.

- Cellular Medicine provides the scientific rationale explaining why all these conditions are closely related to deficiencies in essential nutrients. Logically, optimum daily intake of vitamins and other essential nutrients is a basic measure to prevent and to correct these health conditions.

The Cardiovascular System
Is Composed of Millions of Cells

Blood Vessel Wall Cells

Blood Cells

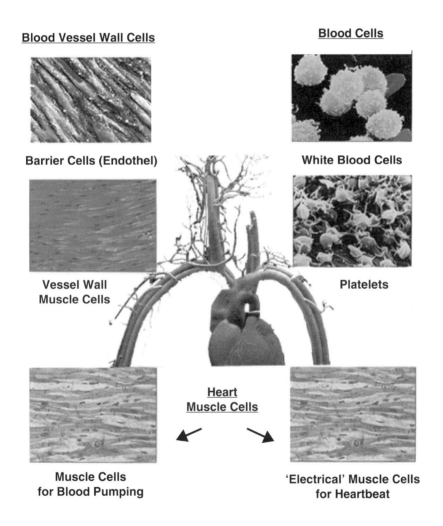

Barrier Cells (Endothel)

White Blood Cells

Vessel Wall
Muscle Cells

Platelets

Heart
Muscle Cells

Muscle Cells
for Blood Pumping

'Electrical' Muscle Cells
for Heartbeat

Deficiencies of Essential Nutrients
in Millions of *Heart Muscle Cells* Contribute to
Irregular Heartbeat and Heart Failure

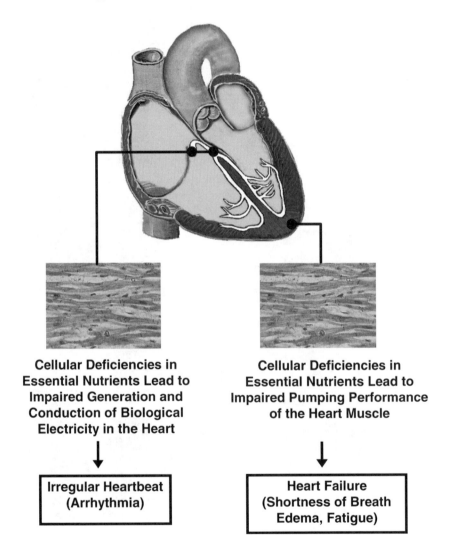

Cellular Deficiencies in Essential Nutrients Lead to Impaired Generation and Conduction of Biological Electricity in the Heart

↓

Irregular Heartbeat (Arrhythmia)

Cellular Deficiencies in Essential Nutrients Lead to Impaired Pumping Performance of the Heart Muscle

↓

Heart Failure (Shortness of Breath Edema, Fatigue)

Deficiencies of Essential Nutrients
in Millions of *Vascular Wall Cells* Contribute to
High Blood Pressure and Atherosclerosis

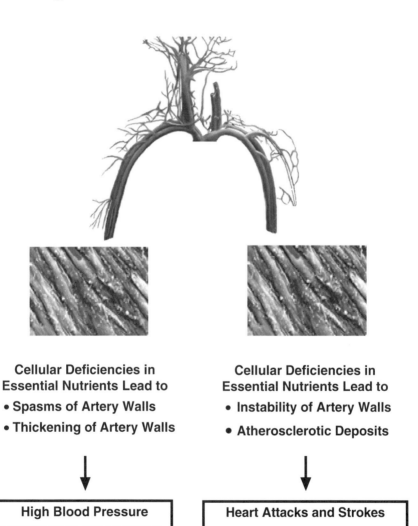

**Cellular Deficiencies in
Essential Nutrients Lead to**

- **Spasms of Artery Walls**
- **Thickening of Artery Walls**

**Cellular Deficiencies in
Essential Nutrients Lead to**

- **Instability of Artery Walls**
- **Atherosclerotic Deposits**

High Blood Pressure

Heart Attacks and Strokes

Cellular Medicine -

Breakthrough for Patients With Coronary Heart Disease

The Facts About Coronary Heart Disease

- **Over ten million Americans** are currently diagnosed with coronary heart disease (leading to heart attacks) or cerebrovascular disease (leading to strokes). The epidemic spread of these cardiovascular diseases is largely due to the fact that until now the most important causes of coronary heart disease and atherosclerosis have been insufficiently or not at all understood.

- **Conventional Medicine** is largely confined to treating the *symptoms* of this disease. Calcium antagonists, betablockers, nitrates and other drugs are prescribed to alleviate angina pain. Surgical procedures (angioplasty, bypass surgery) are applied to improve blood flow mechanically. Hardly any conventional treatment targets the underlying problem - the instability of the vascular wall triggering the development of atherosclerotic deposits.

- **Cellular Medicine provides a breakthrough in our understanding of the cause of coronary heart disease.** The primary cause of coronary heart disease and other forms of atherosclerotic cardiovascular disease is a chronic deficiency in vitamins and other essential nutrients in millions of cells that compose the vascular wall. This leads to instability of the vascular walls, to lesions and cracks, to atherosclerotic deposits and eventually to heart attacks or strokes. Since the primary cause of cardiovascular disease is a deficiency of essential nutrients in the vascular wall, a daily optimum intake of these essential nutrients is the primary measure to prevent atherosclerosis and to help repair damage that has already occurred.

- **Scientific research and clinical studies** have already documented the particular value of vitamin C, vitamin E, beta carotene and of the natural amino acids lysine and proline in the prevention of cardiovascular disease and in improving the health of patients with existing cardiovascular disease.

- **America's Most Successful Cardiovascular Health Program** comprises selected essential nutrients to help prevent cardiovascular disease naturally and to help repair already existing damage. The following pages document health improvements from patients with coronary heart disease and other forms of cardiovascular disease who have greatly benefited from this program.

- **My recommendation for patients**: Start immediately with this program and inform your doctor about it. Take the essential nutrients *in addition to* your regular medication. Do not stop your regular medication without consulting your doctor. Document your health improvements with this natural program.

Coronary Artery Disease (Angina Pectoris)
Other Forms of Atherosclerotic Cardiovascular Disease

Primary Cause:

**Basic Prevention
and Basic Correction:**

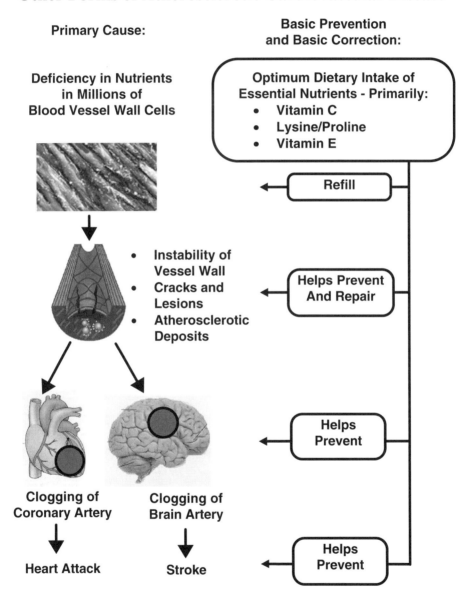

**Deficiency in Nutrients
in Millions of
Blood Vessel Wall Cells**

**Optimum Dietary Intake of
Essential Nutrients - Primarily:**
- **Vitamin C**
- **Lysine/Proline**
- **Vitamin E**

Refill

- **Instability of
Vessel Wall**
- **Cracks and
Lesions**
- **Atherosclerotic
Deposits**

**Helps Prevent
And Repair**

**Helps
Prevent**

**Clogging of
Coronary Artery**

**Clogging of
Brain Artery**

Heart Attack

Stroke

**Helps
Prevent**

27

Dear Dr. Rath:

*I am a 57 year old male who had a heart attack on November 20, 1986. I was told by my cardiologist that I had incurred **a myocardial infarction** of a small artery in the lower portion of my heart. It was determined that angioplasty or some other surgical procedure was not relevant or pertinent. The after effects were **reduced energy and stamina, angina pectoris and other related symptoms** typical to this condition. Since that time, I have been on a calcium antagonist medication.*

Follow up angioplasty procedures were performed in October 1987 and February 1993. Evidence of noticeable change in my condition was limited to some increase in the partial blockage in other major coronary arteries.

I began following your cardiovascular health program last October. This April another angioplasty was performed on me

(continued)

by a cardiologist who is highly respected and has many years of experience in this specialty area. He has performed several thousand of these procedures; however, he was amazed at what he observed in my case.

He found the previously blocked artery to have 25% to 30% blood flow and no advancement in the partial obstruction of other arteries. *His comment was, "Your arteries look great, I don't know what you are doing, but keep doing it." He further commented that this was only the second time he had observed an artery opening up that was previously blocked, without some surgical procedure.*

*I have experienced remarkable improvement in my general health through a **reduction in the incidence of angina, chest pressure, shortness of breath and increased energy and endurance**. I truly believe your cardiovascular health program will extend my life and eliminate what appeared to the inevitable need for cardiac by-pass surgery some time in the future. Your program has dramatically improved my life and I am very grateful.*

Sincerely,   *L.T.*

Dear Dr. Rath:

*In June 1994 I was taken to the emergency room of a hospital with severe chest pains - the EKG showed my heart was strong, but with an invasive test through my arteries they discovered a **20% blockage in an artery leading to my heart**. Also with a sonogram they found a 40% blockage in an artery in my shoulder leading to my brain. I also had an arrhythmia.*

A month later, it was discovered by a cat-scan that I had cancer in one kidney. I had the kidney removed, my first major operation.

*From July until January I was unable to recover from this operation. **I was always out of breath, tired, no stamina, no pep.** It was proven by catscan that I was free of cancer.*

Three doctors could not answer why I was tired - out of breath - no endurance.

I found your book in a health food store. The owner recommended I read it and start on your cardiovascular health program. These vitamins were designed to fulfill your requirements that you outline in your book.

(continued)

__Within 2 weeks I regained my strength, pep, breath and well on my way to regaining my endurance.__ I also am on a program of better diet and physical therapy; however, I credit this miraculous, speedy recovery to the vitamins you recommend in your book.

You may use this letter as testimony as you wish. Thank you for your efforts. Everyone should be made aware of your discoveries.

Thanks to your efforts and discoveries, I am on my way to full health and fitness again.

Sincerely,   *H.K.*

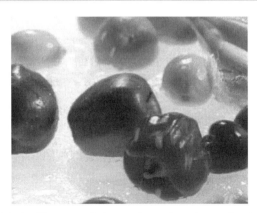

Apples are high in fiber, pectin's, various vitamins and minerals such as vitamin C, vitamin A, potassium, calcium, magnesium and phosphorus.

Dear Dr. Rath:

In mid-January I began experiencing some intermittent discomfort in the muscles of the left arm and shoulder. As the pain increased, I thought it was either a pinched nerve or a heart problem. I went to a physician for diagnosis (stress test, EKG, etc.). The EKG displayed an inverted T wave. I was whisked to a hospital and received angioplastic surgery.

*I was told the Lateral Anterior Descending **artery was 95% blocked** and that another artery, unspecified, was 40% blocked. After release from the hospital, I was told that blockage had reoccurred and asked if I wanted to repeat the procedure. My answer: No. I received a prescription for medication and advised to take aspirin also.*

There has been no reoccurrence of pain, but a mild intermittent tingling sensation occurred in the left arm and hand during February and March. Then I started your cardiovascular health program. I have been taking L-Lysine and vitamin C (700 mg Lysine & 500 mg vitamin C) three times a day.

(continued)

***There has been improvement I experience neither pain nor tingling now.** I do believe your cardiovascular health program has been central in restoring the circulatory system to health*

Yours truly,   *H.M.*

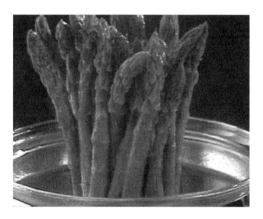

Asparagus is nutrient rich and a good source of vitamin C, vitamin A, sulfur, folic acid and potassium.

Dear Dr. Rath:

A friend of mine started on your program a few weeks ago because of minor heart problems. I did not know, but he was also **scheduled for eye surgery because of blood vessel blockage**. *He went into the hospital for surgery last week and the doctor looked into his eyes and couldn't believe what he saw.* **His blockages had cleared and he no longer needed the surgery done!** *This was only a few weeks of use and nothing else had been changed. Needless to say he has been telling everyone he knows about your cardiovascular health program.*

Sincerely,   *C.Z.*

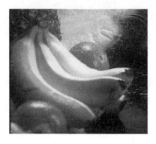

Bananas are a good source of potassium. They also contain various other important nutrients such as carbohydrates, iron, selenium and magnesium.

Dear Dr. Rath:

The patient is an eighty-five year old woman who was diagnosed in 1985 with angina pectoris. She was told by the doctor that **_two major arteries were 95% blocked_**.

The doctor prescribed nitroglycerin tablets to relieve the painful condition induced by stress. She has been taking 3 to 4 nitroglycerin tablets a day for her chest pain for 10 years.

Last December she started to follow your cardiovascular health program. **_After two months she was almost completely off the nitroglycerin tablets and now only occasionally takes one._**

Sincerely,   *R.A.*

Dear Dr. Rath:

*I am 57 year old man and have lived a very active life. **Two years ago I was diagnosed with angina pectoris**, the cardiologist prescribed a calcium antagonist and nitroglycerin tablets, as needed for pain. Dr. Rath, I was taking 8 to 10 nitroglycerin tablets weekly every time I attempted to do anything strenuous or I got the slightest agitated, I needed one.*

*I was introduced to your cardiovascular health program and a fiber formula and **within 6 weeks I no longer needed the nitroglycerin**. I was not able to mow my yard with a push mower without stopping every 5 to 10 minutes and take a nitroglycerin tablet. About a week ago I push mowed, edged and weeded my entire yard, about three hours work and did not stop at all and did not have any chest pain. I felt great.*

*I have also lost about 10 pounds and my cholesterol level dropped from 274 to 191 and still going down. **My doctor says he is real pleased with my condition**.*

(continued)

I am indebted to you for a great change in my life. I did not have insurance for the $15,000 in hospital and doctor's bills.

With your help I will be able to live a more fulfilling life for a longer time for a lot less money.

Thank you so very much,   *H.D.*

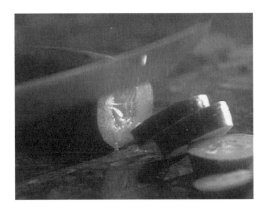

Cucumbers are low in calories, their seeds have plenty of vitamin E. Cucumbers have some vitamin A, vitamin C also potassium and other minerals.

Dear Dr. Rath:

*Last June I was diagnosed for an **unstable angina pectoris due to coronary atherosclerosis.** In order to obtain the best diagnostic and prognostic information, I agreed to undergo a coronary angiogram. The study found single vessel disease in the form of a short 99% stenosis of the large first obtuse marginal branch and a short 50-70% stenosis of the circumflex artery. A balloon coronary angioplasty was recommended, but I decided to go on a medical program instead. I was able to tolerate the problem and decided that I have to live with it.*

*Five months ago I was introduced to your cardiovascular health program. In all honesty, I have had nothing but excellent results! **My doctor has reduced the amount of medicine I was taking, I walk at least four miles a day, and my angina just seems to have disappeared**. I am 68 years old, and I wish I would have known about your program earlier, as I am sure that my problem could have been prevented.*

I cannot thank my nephew enough for introducing me to your cardiovascular health program — I know I will use it as long as I live.

Kindest regards,   *B.S.*

Dear Dr. Rath,

Since following your cardiovascular health program on a regular basis, I am happy to report a very significant increase in my general energy level. My physical and mental health seems to be enjoying increased vitality. **I have no present indications of angina,** *and my ability to walk vigorously including a climb around the hills that are in my neighborhood is most encouraging.* **No huffing and puffing and pausing to catch my breath, as before.**

I am able to walk around my neighborhood hills without interrupting the rhythm and flow of my conversation. This too is an apparent and welcome change from the days before I followed your program. I also pursue a very modest weight loss program, eating much less than before — with no loss of energy. I feel that your program is most significant in all this, and I am happy to share my views with you and anyone who might benefit from them.

Sincerely yours, *R.A.*

Dear Dr. Rath:

*In January of this year I began experiencing chest pains when exercising. In April my doctor told me, on the basis of an EKG, that **I had suffered a heart attack**. He continued prescribing a betablocker which I had been taking for high blood pressure for many years.*

In May I started following your cardiovascular health program and also went on a very strict vegetarian, no-fat diet. My chest pain during exercise began to lessen after just two weeks of this regimen.

***I have now been on a diet and your program for 2 months, and I now have no chest pain or breathlessness at all, even when cycling or walking energetically for several hours at a time**. I also feel better than I have felt for years, with lots of energy and high spirits. My confidence level in my heart condition is so good that I no longer carry nitroglycerin pills with me when setting out on a bicycle ride or a walk. I feel young and bright, and I look great. People I run into say how good I look.*

(continued)

Since the only change in my lifestyle has been your cardiovascular health program and diet, I have to say that one or both of these factors have caused this dramatic change in my health.

For what it is worth, I tend to think that the combination of both these factors together is what has caused my health to improve.

Yours truly,   *K.P.*

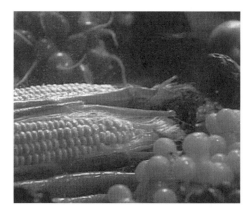

Corn is rich in energy generating starch and complex carbohydrates, fiber, protein, B-vitamins and minerals. Fresh corn contains vitamin C, folic acid, and lots of potassium and magnesium.

Dear Dr. Rath,

I am so happy to tell you the wonderful story of the use of your cardiovascular health program and how I feel that it has saved my life.

*Last September I had gone to the university to watch a football game and could not make it up the steps in the stadium despite wearing a nitroglycerin patch, and by October last year **I could not walk 100 yards without the pain of angina.***

*I found out about your discovery and took it triple strength four times a day for three weeks and **by Thanksgiving I had forgotten I had a heart problem**. Now, in July of this year I am working without pain and feeling super! Too bad you did not have the patent before I had undergone two bypass surgeries.*

Thanks for More Life,   *J.G.*

Health improvement in eighty-five year old woman.

Ten years ago __she was diagnosed with angina pectoris__. She was told by the doctor that two major arteries were 95% blocked.

The doctor prescribed nitroglycerin tablets to relieve the painful condition induced by stress. She has been taking three nitroglycerin tablets a day for her chest pains for 10 years.

Last December she started on your cardiovascular health program. __After two months she was almost completely off nitroglycerin__. She now takes a nitroglycerin tablet only occasionally.

Sincerely,   D.H.

Dear Dr. Rath:

*I started following your cardiovascular health program last August after I was diagnosed as having severe heart disease. **I had angina for 8 years**.*

*Now, nearly a year later, I feel fine and have very slight angina infrequently, plus I walk 3.6 miles daily and **don't have any restrictions**.*

Sincerely,   *M.B.*

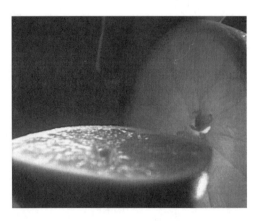

Grapefruits help to improve digestion and utilization of foods. They are low in calories but rich in vitamin C as well as potassium.

Dear Dr. Rath:

My dad was diagnosed with blockages of the heart in October last year. He also suffered from the pains of Angina and from arrhythmia.

Dad could not walk a block without concern for his ability to make it home again *(because of the fatigue in his legs). And when he had blood work done, it was with great difficulty that the medical technicians collected blood samples.*

*My dad was concerned for his life and because he **had two ischemic events** (four years ago) along with being diabetic and being eighty years of age, his team of medical devisors ruled out an invasive procedure as a remedy.*

When I was first made aware of your breakthrough non-invasive therapy, I could not believe our good fortune. Immediately we placed dad on your cardiovascular health program. Within a day he reported good results. "I feel good!" was his response after the first day.

(continued)

The second day he told me that his energy level had increased significantly. "I was able to work in the garage all day today without getting tired!"

The third day and dad had walked a block and returned without difficulty - no pains, fatigue or apprehension.

The chest pains went away by December, and in January, on our way to the cardiologist's office, dad, having forgotten his essential nutrients for his doctors' inspection and review, ran back into the house (well, trotted anyway) to retrieve them. I got so excited by the event that I immediately started calling people on my car phone to share with them what I had just witnessed - a miracle!

My dad's heart no longer skips a beat, his angina is gone, *his blood flows freely when he proudly donates blood samples. His doctors are amazed with his newfound state of health. And we are very, very happy.*

Last week my dad took a ten block walk without difficulty; he is proud and grateful.

Thank you, Dr. Rath. Your research has given my dad back his life.

Sincerely,   *M.T.*

Dear Dr. Rath:

Your cardiovascular health program has done so much to improve the quality of my life, healthwise, that I would like to share it with others.

I was 83 years old last February. ___I was having so much angina pain that my family doctor sent me to a cardiologist, who did an angioplasty___*. In the meantime my 78 year old husband had triple by-pass followed by a stroke. I had to get better to take care of him, but I continued to have the same pains.*

A second cardiologist did angioplasty in August last year which did not help, so in September I had a double by-pass, needing a third.

My son started me on your cardiovascular health program. In January of this year I was still having angina, due to an artery they were unable to by-pass. ___After 3 months I quit having pains, due to stress or strain or excitement and now, after six months, I feel great and do almost as much physically as I did 5 or 10 years ago.___

(continued)

My husband, although hampered by his stroke, also enjoys better health with your cardiovascular health program.

Sincerely,   *L.W.*

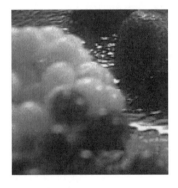

Grapes are high in fructose and fiber. They also contain a good amount of vitamin A, vitamin C, B-vitamins, potassium and other minerals.

Dear Dr. Rath:

*I was very excited about the possibility of improving heart function and reversing heart disease due to atherosclerosis after reading your two books this past February. **I have familial hypercholesterolemia and had a myocardial infarction six years ago at age 40. Your theories made sense to me, and I was determined to put them to the test, as my efforts through dietary modifications over the last few years proved fruitless**. My career in medical sales is stress filled and leaves little time for physical exercise.*

*I started following your cardiovascular health program in February this year, along with a fiber formula. Within the first month I started feeling less tired and was able to keep on going without exhaustion or angina. **Within two months the pain in my lower left leg due to poor circulation (atherosclerosis) disappeared**. My heart feels like it's just on overdrive - just purring along - no longer pounding in my chest.*

My annual physical in May was quite interesting. I never told my doctor I was doing anything different, but he shared with me that my EKG looked normal!

(continued)

I guess you could say that this was objective proof that my subjective observations are very real.

I asked my doctor about possibly lowering my heart medication (calcium antagonist, betablocker). **_He said that, based on my examination, he would take me off all this medicine_** *if I lost 17 more pounds of weight. I had already lost 12 pounds since February, so I see losing 17 pounds just a matter of time. My goal is to get to my target weight by the end of September.*

I have supplemented your cardiovascular health program with additional vitamin C, L-proline, and L-lysine. I do not know if my atherosclerosis will ever be 100% reversed, but I do know that whatever progress your program has done for me so far has already **_improved my condition and has impacted my overall quality of life_**. *I will continue your cardiovascular health program the rest of my life, and recommend it to any concerned about their health. I thank God for your research.*

Sincerest regards,   *R.R.*

Dear Dr. Rath:

I am writing this letter to you with thanks for your wonderful cardiovascular health program. I appreciate the many hours of dedication that you have placed within your research in order to eradicate heart disease.

Your program has personally touched my family. **_My mother had been diagnosed several years ago with angina pectoris_**. *Last November she began your program.*

Within six weeks the pains in her heart as well as some undiagnosed pains in her stomach disappeared. *While experiencing these constant pains she had become very fearful and depressed. Once the pains lifted she felt new hope, began walking, and stated that her breathing was much easier.*

The impact of her better health has reverberated through our family. She is happy and her sense of humor has returned.

(continued)

Due to the family history of heart disease I started following your cardiovascular health program last November, also. Although I had no diagnosed heart problems I feel a level of comfort in knowing I am doing preventive health maintenance that should ensure not having the same problems my mother has endured.

I cannot thank you enough for all you have done for my mother and our family.

Sincerely,   *K.S.*

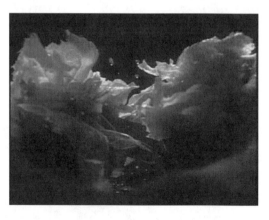

Lettuce is rich in vitamin A, vitamin C, folic acid, calcium, potassium and iron.

Dear Dr. Rath:

I started your cardiovascular health program four months ago. I had been suffering with angina pectoris pains and wearing a nitroglycerin patch for 6 months prior to starting your program. After six days I noticed the pain/strain in my chest was less severe, but the headaches for 6 or more hours were still present while I had the nitroglycerin-patch on.

<u>On the 7th day I took the nitroglycerin patch off because of the severe headaches and what I found was the pulling/strain in my chest was non-existent and absolutely no headaches</u>.

After the 7th day I continued to carry the nitroglycerin patch in my pocket, but did not put it on. I carried the patch in my pocket for 2 months, then stopped carrying it.

In April I told my doctor about how well I felt and that I had stopped using the patch. I gave my doctor a brochure describing your cardiovascular health program. In May I saw him again and told him how great I felt because of your program.

Sincerely,   *D.*

Dear Dr. Rath:

*My father is a **72 year old man with coronary artery disease**. In 1988 he had 3 vessel coronary artery bypass and had a silent myocardial infarction some time prior to surgery. In December 1994 he had a routine stress test, which he failed. At that time he started to take double the essential nutrients recommended in your cardiovascular health program. **After 5 weeks a thallium stress test was performed, which he passed**. I'm including both stress test results.*

In addition, my father has been suffering from a chronic controlled atrial fibrillation since his surgery in 1988. He takes digitalis medication and a betablocker. In March of 1995 he also underwent surgery for an aortic aneurysm. Surgery was uneventful and he is recovering well. He continues to follow your program and continues on his other medications.

Since starting your cardiovascular health program I see my father less anxious about the failed stress test and more confident he won't have to go through cardiac surgery again. The first time was a difficult experience.

God bless you in your work,   *A.J.*

Dear Dr. Rath:

*I am 47 years old and have **<u>severe coronary calcification</u>** and multiple lesions scattered throughout the heart - some areas 80-90% blocked. I am unable to have open heart surgery or any other procedure. I've had this condition for 9 years.*

*I take several prescription medications. **<u>For ten months I have been following your cardiovascular health program and I observe less angina, higher HDL and lower LDL blood levels.</u>***

I feel a lot better now than ten months ago. I also seem to have more energy.

Sincerely,   *M.D.*

Dear Dr. Rath:

*I had been having **chest pain (angina pectoris) for several years** on the average of about every three weeks.*

Since I started your cardiovascular health program over 90 days ago, I have only had chest pain one time, which was about three weeks after starting your program.

I feel that proper nutrition can prevent eighty percent of our health problems.

Sincerely,   *B.T.*

Health improvement in 54 year old man:

He had chest pains and pain in left arm for 6 months. His doctor advised a stress test and a possible angiogram.

After 45 days on your cardiovascular health program these symptoms disappeared. *He also has more energy than he had before.*

Sincerely, *J.L.*

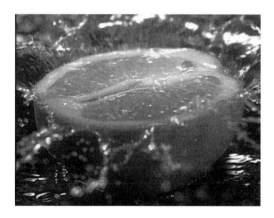

One glass of orange juice provides about 125 mg of vitamin C.
Oranges contain almost all the vitamins and minerals.

Dear Dr. Rath:

*I am happy to write to you telling you of the benefits that I have received since starting your cardiovascular health program. It has been approximately one month since I began and I have been able to notice a **remarkable improvement in my energy and vitality**. Several of my neighbors have commented that I look better than I have for years.*

It was a little over three years ago that I suffered a brain-stem stroke which has left me with a little disability in my walking and some weakness. However since that time I have had surgery for a narrowing of the arteries (endarterectomy). Recovery from that surgery was uneventful. Then in 1992 I developed a blood disorder with low platelets (down to 3,000). Treatment has been extensive including chemotherapy, blood infusions, and even a splenectomy. A complication to all of this was blood clots in both legs. It appears that all is beginning to turn around and a lab report just today showed that my platelets have gone up to 38,000. I believe that this program is having a marked effect on my getting better.

Sincerely,   *G.S.*

Dear Dr. Rath:

*I read your book, "Eradicating Heart Disease" about a year ago when I was told I had severe blockage of the coronary arteries, and I had a **triple bypass operation**. At that time I started following your cardiovascular health program. All of my checkups since my surgery have been outstanding. **I attribute much of the good news to your program**.*

For a long time I have maintained an opinion that there was a better answer to heart disease than the standard American Medical Association medical approach. Thank you for finding the answer and making it available to all of us who need it.

I recently subscribed to your "Health Now" newsletter.

Sincerely,   *C.S.*

Dear Dr. Rath:

I offer this letter as support for your testimonials on the cardiovascular health program.

*I was born prematurely with a hematoma that doctors treated with penicillin and radiation at age 3 months. Little did I know what was in store for me later in life! I had wonderful parents who nursed me through normal childhood diseases who felt helpless to aid me when I developed cancer. Who know what particular stress or carcinogen finally triggered this abnormal process in motion. I underwent a mastectomy, **aggressive chemotherapy,** a reconstruction, and then in 1993 learned my cancer was still with me. Doctors had misjudged the margin and cancer was still under my pectoralis muscle. Radiation followed which left my lungs and heart weakened, but the cancer was in remission.*

Now at age 42 after facing a miscarriage, mastectomy, and sadly a divorce all within a year of each other. . . I was unwilling to succumb to the fear of death! I began an intense study of my body's immune system

(continued)

nutrition, and homeopathy, disparate to find a natural way to cope with the unpleasant side effects from the medication I would be for the rest of my life.

In 1994 a business colleague and friend introduced me to your cardiovascular health program and other preventive health care measures. ***The side effects I had indicated the beginnings of cardiovascular or circulatory problems.*** *Leg cramps and tingling fingers and toes would keep me awake at night and terrible hot flashes would disturb me many times daily. I was short of breath at the least little exertion and ate needlessly to handle stress.*

I am happy to report that ***the side effects disappeared after four months of steady use of your cardiovascular health program and related natural measures****. I believe that they were critical to the support and strength of my immune system and were responsible for the decrease in the circulatory problems. I have added critical fiber to my diet; my blood sugar levels have stabilized; and my cholesterol dropped from 189 to 155. I feel wonderful!*

Sincerely,   *K.M.*

Dear Dr. Rath,

A health care worker for eleven years, I've seen a lot of patients with cardiovascular disease. As a matter of fact, the patient I have now has gone through a series of operations for cardiovascular disease. Her condition gave me a look at what I could become if I didn't take care of my health.

*The greatest day of my life was when I was introduced to your cardiovascular health program. Within two months a **tremendous change in my health occurred.***

On my right foot, the middle toe was numb, no feeling, no life. Today there is feeling there. Tingling, a good feeling. Also my legs don't hurt anymore. Moreover, my eyesight is clearer.

What more can I say. Your cardiovascular health program is the greatest health program I have experienced. What I like more is that it is all natural.

Keep up the good work,   *D.S.*

Dear Dr. Rath,

Thank you for your cardiovascular health program. **_I have found it has helped my circulation._**

I usually spend most of January and February and even parts of March each year working in my woodwork shop, a separate building with a cold wood floor. I would end up with very cold feet, to the point where when I came in to the house for lunch, I would put my insulated boots in the sun too warm and not go back out till my feet were warm.

This past winter my feet were warm all the time, even going to bed. What a difference!

My father had such pain in his feet from poor circulation the doctor threatened to amputate. I feel this will never be a problem for me.

Thank you for all your research and work in our behalf. It is a blessing to us.

Sincerely,   J.G.

Cellular Medicine -

Breakthrough for Arrhythmia Patients

The Facts About Irregular Heartbeat (Arrhythmia)

- **More than eight million Americans** are currently suffering from irregular heartbeat. Worldwide over one hundred million people suffer from this condition. The epidemic spread of this disease is largely due to the fact that until now the causes of arrhythmia have been insufficiently or not at all understood. In some cases arrhythmias are the result of a heart attack; in most cases, however, they develop without any prior cardiac event.

- **Conventional Medicine** is largely confined to treating the *symptoms* of this disease. Betablockers and many other antiarrhytmic drugs target the symptoms of irregular heartbeat, not its underlying cause.

- **Cellular Medicine provides a breakthrough in our understanding of the causes of irregular heartbeat**. Arrhythmias are frequently caused or aggravated by deficiencies of certain vitamins and other essential nutrients in millions of electrical muscle cells of the heart. These cells are responsible for generation and conduction of biological electricity needed for a regular heartbeat. Deficiencies of vitamins and other essential nutrients impair the function of theses cells, frequently resulting in irregular heartbeat.

- **Scientific research and clinical studies** have already documented the particular value of magnesium, carnitine, and other essential nutrients in helping to normalize different types of irregular heartbeat, thereby improving the quality of life for patients with arrhythmia.

- **America's Most Successful Cardiovascular Health Program** comprises selected essential nutrients which are needed for optimum function of millions of cells, including the electrical muscle cells of the heart. The following pages document health improvements from arrhythmia patients who have greatly benefited from this program.

- **My recommendations for arrhythmia patients**: Start immediately with this program and inform your doctor about it. Take the essential nutrients *in addition to* your regular medication. Do not stop your regular medication without consulting your doctor. Document your health improvements with this natural program.

Irregular Heartbeat

Frequent Cause:

**Basic Prevention
and Basic Correction:**

**Deficiency of Essential Nutrients
in Millions of *Electrical* Heart
Muscle Cells**

**Optimum Dietary Intake of
Essential Nutrients Primarily**
- **Vitamin C**
- **Magnesium**
- **Coenzyme-Q-10**

Refill

**Insufficient Generation
or Conduction
of Cellular Electricity
in Electrical
Heart Muscle Cells**

**Helps Prevent
and Correct**

Normal   **Deficient**

**Irregular
Contraction
of the Heart**

**Helps Prevent
and Correct**

**Helps Prevent
and Correct**

Arrhythmia

Dear Dr. Rath:

I am 54 years of age and have had a very **irregular heartbeat for at least 20 years**. *This was diagnosed as second degree electrical heart block.*

I have never taken any medication for this. I have had a stress test done approximately every 2 years and the heart block showed up on the EKG. I was told that as long as my heartbeat becomes regular when I exercised that I did not need any other treatment.

I do not have any other circulatory problems and I am very fit for my age. For the last 20 years I have jogged, played tennis and eat a low fat high fiber diet.

I started your cardiovascular health program this year, and by mid February I noticed that my heartbeat was regular when at rest.

(continued)

In June I even went back to the doctor where I had my last EKG done so there would be a basis for comparison. **_The doctor found that there was no longer any arrhythmia seen. I have enclosed a copy of his report_**.

I am sure that your cardiovascular health program is responsible for the correction of my irregular heartbeat, as I had not changed my lifestyle in any other respect.

Sincerely,   *T.H.*

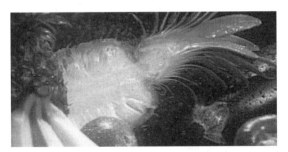

One cup of pineapples supplies 2.5 mg of manganese, it is also rich in vitamin A, vitamin C, and potassium. Pineapples also contain a digestive enzyme, bromelain, that helps to optimize digestion.

Dear Dr. Rath:

*I wanted to thank you for your research and for your cardiovascular health program. **<u>After three weeks of the program I am no longer experiencing chest pain.</u>***

With my family cardiovascular history, both of my parents experienced heart attacks before they were 30 years old - the pains were concerning me. I am 34 years old now and have a mitral valve prolapse. I have avoided going to prescription medication to this point, but I was afraid I was going to have to begin that form of therapy to relieve my symptoms.

*Now I do not have to go on drugs with all their side effects. **<u>I feel great about your cardiovascular health program and its ability to help me naturally.</u>***

My mother and brother are now on the program also.

Thank you,   *T.W.*

Dear Dr. Rath:

Thank you for developing your cardiovascular health program, which I am currently following. Several years ago I was diagnosed as having **Hyperkinetic Heart Syndrome**. *I took medication for a few years, but did not like how I felt — too slowed down and not able to respond quickly to physical exertion.*

During times of great stress, I would have pounding, irregular, racing heartbeats at nighttime when I am trying to fall asleep. Also, when confronted with a stressful encounter during the day, my heart would immediately jump into a racing, pounding episode. I heard your lecture in May. I immediately read two of your books "Why Animals Don't Get Heart Attacks" and "Eradicating Heart Disease".

A week later I began following your cardiovascular health program **and within a few days, I was no longer experiencing pounding, irregular, racing heartbeats** *at bedtime.*

(continued)

Within a week I noticed that when confronted with a stressful encounter during the day, my heart did not jump into racing and pounding episode.

I have taken vitamin, mineral, herbal supplements for several years, but have never had this amazing result before now! Thank you so very much!

Yours truly,   *C.M.*

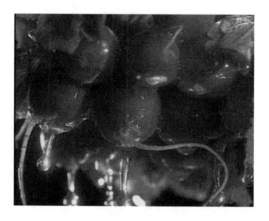

Radishes are rich in vitamin C, folic acid and most of the trace minerals (iron, zinc, silicon).

Dear Dr. Rath:

In February I introduced my 74 year old grandmother to your cardiovascular health program. ***Her slow and irregular heart beat had led her doctor to begin preliminary preparations to install a pacemaker.***

After about three weeks on your program her heart action was sufficiently improved to cause the doctor to postpone this procedure*.*

This lady is now a faithful follower of your cardiovascular health program and, although she faces other medical challenges, her heart condition continues to improve, and the use of a pacemaker is no longer being considered.

Sincerely,   *K.C.*

Dear Dr. Rath:

*I wanted you to know that **for the last three years, I have had abnormal EKG's**. I went through all the cardiac testing and was diagnosed with damaged areas in my heart and with a weak heart muscle.*

I have been on your cardiovascular health program for four months, my EKG is now totally normal.

I highly recommend your program to anyone who has cardiac problems.

Sincerely,   *L.H.*

Dear. Dr. Rath:

I am excited to tell you of my experience.

*I am a 60 year old female who has fought hypertension for the past 20 years with many different types of medications which would work for a while, then become ineffective and start giving me problems. In November of 1993 new symptoms began for which I was referred to a cardiologist who determined I was well on my way to a pacemaker. He decided not to treat this aggressively, but instead, through medication. I have avoided surgery. In February of this year **I began experiencing prolonged bouts of tachycardia**, and was prescribed new, additional medication.*

*In March I was introduced to your cardiovascular health program. Although I was skeptical, I decided to give it a try. I've just started my third month on your program and have been able to reduce my blood pressure medication by one-third. **The episodes of tachycardia have decreased dramatically, both in intensity and duration.**￼*

(continued)

75

If an episode occurs, it is almost insignificant. At the same time, I have also noted a dramatic effect in that my ankles are no longer swelling at the end of a work day.

Following my last lab work, my doctor told me "Your numbers look like someone one-half your age."

Needless to say I am a staunch believer in your cardiovascular health program.

Sincerely,   *F.S.*

Dear Dr. Rath:

*Two months ago I was **experiencing loud heartbeats, tachycardia and irregular beating of the heart**. I saw my doctor who promptly put me on an anti-arrhythmic drug. I can honestly say the medication did me absolutely no good.*

*Then, I started to follow your cardiovascular health program. What a smart decision that was! **Within a few days, the tachycardia stopped and I've not experienced any loud or irregular heartbeats**. It's like a miracle.*

It must be the combination of nutrients in your program because I had been taking Coenzyme Q10 separately from my regular vitamins. I tell everyone I know about the benefits of your program.

Because of your research, I'm able to continue working.

Sincerely,   *B.M.*

Dear Dr. Rath,

*Thank you for your research and dedication for the reversal of heart disease. I cannot thank you enough. **<u>I have had irregular heart beat, racing rhythm, and sometimes my heart would skip a beat</u>**. My cardiovascular system is not the best. My father has had bypass surgery, and I have had veins removed. I want to tell you emphatically that **<u>since I have been on your cardiovascular health program, my heart beat has been regular -- no missing beats -- no racing beats</u>**. I have had the irregular heart beat for years and the racing and skip beating about one and one-half years. I have taken no medication for this, as I do not like prescription drugs.*

Since I started following your program I feel wonderful, and I know your treatment is helping me.

Thank you, Dr. Rath.

Sincerely,   *M.J.*

Dear Dr. Rath:

How delightful, after following your cardiovascular health program for just 2 months, one notices the absence of irregular heartbeats, and the freedom to breathe freely*. Confidence is restored as one has increased vigor and endurance. In a word, one spends less time thinking about the heart and more time enjoying life.*

Your cardiovascular health program has become the answer for resolving coronary problems.

I am happy to have this opportunity of expressing my gratitude for your advanced medical research and for your cardiovascular health program.

Yours sincerely,   *J.S.*

Dear Dr. Rath:

I am forty years old and the mother of three. My youngest is 3 and a half, so I am a very busy lady.

*A couple years ago I began to notice occasional periods when **my heart would palpitate or beat harder for no apparent reason. I can honestly say I don't seem to experience that now that I'm on your cardiovascular health program.***

Also, I walk 2 and a half miles 5-6 times/week and never have to slow up or rest. This week I made another observation that I can only attribute to your vitamin program, but I don't know whether it makes sense medically. My last two menstrual periods were virtually free of the usual cramping I experience. I hope that will be a regular side effect.

Thank you for this great program. I have recommended it to several of my friends, and my chiropractor (who is also a well-known nutritionist) was very impressed with it.

Sincerely,   *D.K.*

Dear Dr. Rath:

I have been following your cardiovascular health program since last year. **Since six years I have had episodes of irregular heartbeat** *that cause extreme fatigue. These episodes vary, but I was experiencing them approximately two times per week.*

Since starting on your program I have had only two episodes total. *I had previously taken other nutritional products with very little if any help for this condition. Your program has made a significant change in this condition.*

I also frequently have cold hands, especially during winter time, but this past winter this was also much improved.

Sincerely,   *D.H.*

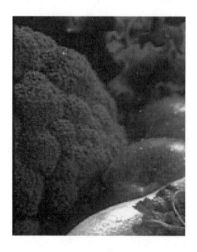

Broccoli is a cruciferous vegetable rich in vitamin A, vitamin C, and folic acid. It is also a good source of potassium, calcium, phosphorus, magnesium, and iron.

Dear Dr. Rath:

I am glad to be able to tell you about my experience with your cardiovascular health program.

*Two years ago in April, I got pregnant and soon after I had a real problem **with my heart pounding** — something that my doctor looked into but couldn't explain, so we assumed it was associated with the pregnancy.*

After my daughter was born in December I expected this to go away but it didn't. I started on your cardiovascular health program last October. I started taking your essential nutrients once a day and later two times a day. I noticed some improvements, but still the condition persisted.

It wasn't until I read the testimonials in your book that I realized I should start taking these essential nutrients three times a day.

(continued)

Before I had really never believed that this would help my condition because I had a doctor tell me that this was not a heart disease, but a common thing that younger women have.

Ten days later I started noticing real improvement even when stressed out or tired, my heart wasn't pounding like before. *This is a tremendous relief and a real life improvement in my health. Thank you. I can truly enjoy time with my two daughters a lot better now.*

Sincerely,   *L.J.*

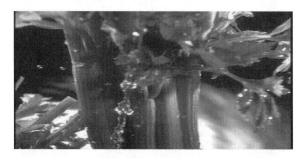

Celery is a good fiber and carbohydrate food with high water content. It is also rich in potassium, calcium, folic acid, vitamin A and C.

Dear Dr. Rath:

I started on your cardiovascular health program last February.

I am a healthy 40 year old male on active duty with the U.S. Navy here in Wash., DC. Up until this point in my life the Navy would not let me donate blood because of arrhythmia.

*<u>**Since three weeks I have no more arrhythmia**</u>. Thank you.*

Sincerely,   *D.G.*

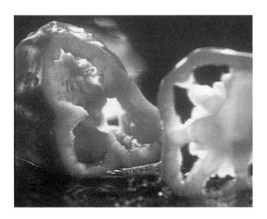

**All peppers are high in vitamin C, bioflavonoids, and vitamin A.
One sweet pepper may have over 500 I.U. of vitamin A
and nearly 150 mg of vitamin C.**

Dear Dr. Rath:

The most important change I've observed since I started following your cardiovascular health program is that which I can only describe as "feeling much better in my body." The two specific improvements are:

I no longer wake up at night with my heart racing and/or beating irregularly.

While I do run out of breath quickly when exerting myself in any way, I no longer feel reluctant to exert my self by walking briskly or up an incline.

So I feel that the daily walking program I've embarked on will soon yield increasing benefits.

You should know I will be 65 in January.

Thank you for your wonderful program,

T.P.

Dear Dr. Rath:

*I have now been following your cardiovascular health program for six months. **I have had atrial fibrillation since 1984**. First I received medication for this condition, followed by electrical cardioversion.*

My heart was in sinus rhythm for one or two months subsequent to that treatment, but then reverted to its initial condition.

*Now, my subjective observations indicate **that my heart rhythm is more regular and that it is sometimes in sinus rhythm**.*

Sincerely yours,   *R.F.*

Dear Dr. Rath:

Before following your cardiovascular health program I used to wake up with a pumping feeling in my chest, no pain, just discomfort. Upon changing position, it would stop.

I no longer have that problem. *I even forget I have a heart. I feel better now than ever in my life. I feel great!*

Sincerely yours,   *J.A.*

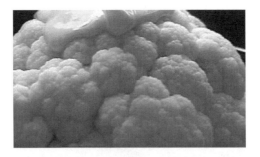

Cauliflower, a member of the highly nutritious cruciferous family, is rich in potassium, folic acid, and vitamin C.

Dear Dr. Rath:

I am a thirty-five year old medical professional. One and one half years ago, due to severe distress to my professional and personal life, I suddenly experienced bouts of **supraventricular tacchycardia which forced me into the emergency room every two months** *over a six month period. My average heart rate would be 230 beats per minute. This condition was life threatening and after my third episode I was referred to the chief of cardiology at the largest hospital in town. After a thorough evaluation, it was concluded that I was not suffering from 'anxiety' but a primary electrical problem with my heart and supraventricular tacchycardia could occur anytime. Therefore, he recommended a surgical procedure called Cardiac Ablation. This procedure involved the insertion of catheters into my subclavian and femoral arteries and threading them to the sinus and atrioventricular nodal regions of the heart and with a DC current, cauterize certain regions of the heart theorized to cause this aberrant electrical circuit.*

(continued)

Although this procedure was definitely indicated, I was too fatigued and weakened from my most recent bout with supra ventricular tacchycardia to consider immediate surgery. I therefore resolved to improve my general health by strengthening myself nutritionally with specific vitamins, minerals, herbal and homeopathic formulas.

*My research lead me to your cardiovascular health program. Your formulation was specific to my health needs and it saved me much time considering I would have purchased many bottles of isolated ingredients that are all found in your program. Therefore, **I embarked on a religious program of supplementation of the essential nutrients you recommend.***

***It has been one and one half years from my last episode.** I have increased energy, little to no chest pain. I look and feel much better. I attribute my success and health to your program.*

Sincerely,   *S.S.*

Cellular Medicine -

Breakthrough for
Heart Failure Patients

The Facts About Heart Failure

- **Millions of Americans** are currently suffering from heart failure resulting in shortness of breath, edema, and fatigue. Worldwide over twenty million people suffer from heart failure conditions and the numbers have tripled over the last four decades. The epidemic spread of this disease is largely due to the fact that until now the causes of heart failure have been insufficiently or not at all understood. In some cases heart failure results after a heart attack; in most cases, such as cardiomyopathies, heart failure develops without any prior cardiac event.

- **Conventional medicine** is largely confined to treating the *symptoms* of heart failure. Diuretic drugs are given to flush out the water that is retained in the body because of the weak pumping function of the heart. In many cases a heart transplant operation is the last resort. Conventional therapies target the symptoms of heart failure - they are largely unable to correct the underlying causes.

- **Cellular medicine provides a breakthrough in our understanding of the causes of heart failure**. Heart failure is frequently caused or aggravated by a deficiency of certain vitamins and other essential nutrients in millions of heart muscle cells. Millions of these muscle cells are responsible for the contraction of the heart muscle and for optimum pumping of blood into the circulation. Deficiencies of vitamins and other essential nutrients impair the pumping performance of the heart, resulting in shortness of breath, edema and fatigue.

- **Scientific research and clinical studies** have already documented the particular value of carnitine, coenzyme Q-10, and other essential nutrients in helping to improve heart performance and the quality of life of heart failure patients.

- **America's Most Successful Cardiovascular Health Program** comprises selected essential nutrients which are needed for optimum function of millions of cells, including the muscle cells of the heart. The following pages document health improvements from heart failure patients who have greatly benefited from this program.

- **My recommendations for heart failure patients**: Start immediately with this program and inform your doctor about it. Take the essential nutrients *in addition to* your regular medication. Do not stop your regular medication without consulting your doctor. Document your health improvements with this natural program.

Heart Failure

Frequent Cause:

**Basic Prevention
and Basic Correction:**

**Deficiency of Essential Nutrients
in Millions of
Heart Muscle Cells**

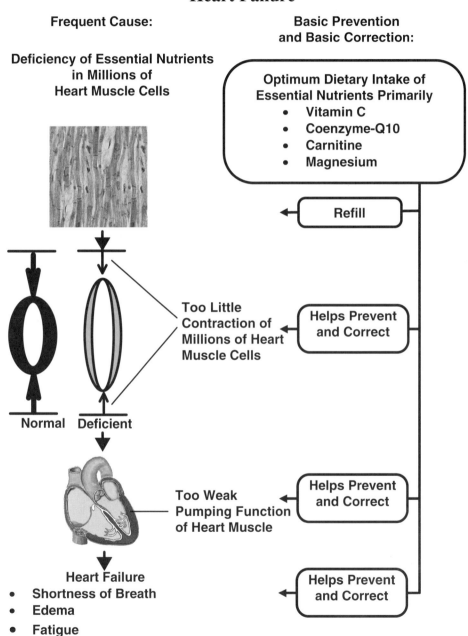

Optimum Dietary Intake of
Essential Nutrients Primarily
- **Vitamin C**
- **Coenzyme-Q10**
- **Carnitine**
- **Magnesium**

Refill

Too Little
Contraction of
Millions of Heart
Muscle Cells

Helps Prevent
and Correct

Normal Deficient

Too Weak
Pumping Function
of Heart Muscle

Helps Prevent
and Correct

Heart Failure
- **Shortness of Breath**
- **Edema**
- **Fatigue**

Helps Prevent
and Correct

Dear Dr. Rath:

My niece is nineteen years old and **has a congenital heart defect**. *Her only hope for survival at birth, the doctors said, was an emergency heart surgery, and we should expect her to die. (I actually made her funeral arrangements for the family).*

But my niece's middle name is "Hope" and she not only survived that first surgery, but five more besides, in addition to other "procedures" and some of these were experimental. From what I understand, she is one of only six other patients in the U.S. who have survived these experimental surgeries to adulthood. Her medical record is like a book. At this point she has so much scar tissue that no other surgeries are considered possible.

(continued)

__My niece has been an invalid much of her life__ - at times playing normally like any other child, but seldom able to finish an entire year of school. __Since her last angioplasty a couple of years ago, she has been in extreme agony and mostly bedridden__.

She did manage last year, by the grace of God and sheer determination, to complete her general education diploma. She walked across the stage (with help and the aid of pain killers) to receive her high school diploma - collapsing on the other side.

Last year she has spent almost entirely in bed, on pain pills and connected to oxygen. The last six months she has required twenty-four hour care, and she's needed help just to get to the potty next to her bed.

In mid-May I called my niece and asked her what her main physical problem was at the moment. She said, gasping, that her greatest difficulty was her breathing, since the main artery between her heart and lungs was plugged. I introduced her to your

(continued)

cardiovascular health program. I said okay, she would try, but she's had a lot of pills and tubes poked into her during her lifetime, and she wasn't really too eager to take more.

*After a few days on your program my niece was becoming very restless and was "all over her bed," even standing up in her bed. Her nurses, who were monitoring the oxygen levels in her blood, asked if she were eating differently or what, because **they noted an increase in the oxygen level.***

***After a month on your cardiovascular health program she was getting out of bed and even fixed herself breakfast and ate it at the kitchen table!** Then she baked her dad a Father's Day cake!*

Near the end of the first month I asked how she was doing. Her normal response to that question is a strained but cheerful, "Oh, I'm doing." This time she said (with great excitement in her voice), "I think it's really working and I'm feeling a lot better."

Well, as you can guess, she continued your cardiovascular health program and she is doing so much better everyone is encouraged.

(continued)

She is even planning to be married! **_She has been out of the house for the first time in over a year_**, and she has been going for rides with her boyfriend on his three-wheel motorcycle, oxygen canister and all!

Today she said **_she had been shopping yesterday for four hours with her fiancé, and didn't even use a wheelchair_**. The oxygen level in her blood, with the oxygen tubes, used to be 96%; now it is 100%.

The entire family and I are very thankful for all your years of study and hard work to come up with this great discovery and to prove it. We thank the Lord that it not only works, but that it is straight from His creation and therefore natural and healthy, without the harmful side effects of drugs.

My niece's heart and lungs are damaged - no question. But at least **_your cardiovascular health program can revitalize what is left and she's not just lying in bed, drugged, sluggish and waiting to die._**

(continued)

To a family who has heard for years: "There is a 99% chance she won't make it," and, "There's nothing more we can do," this program and method could sound like just one more gimmick, but my niece choose to have hope and we are all rejoicing in the results! Thank you.

With sincere gratitude,   *M.A.*

Dear Dr. Rath:

*I started following your cardiovascular health program in January. Since 1989 I have been suffering from **congestive heart failure** and to this day, I am still following the originally prescribed medication with good results. However, I noticed that **I was unable to do any small effort or even walk a couple of blocks without suffering a chest pain** and had to alleviate its intensity by ingesting a tablet.*

It was usual for me to take 3 to 5 tablets per 24 hours, the pain would surface sometimes with no apparent reason.

***After only four months on your program I not only rarely use the nitroglycerin tablets, but I am walking 1.1 mile every morning at a brisk pace, no shortness of breath, no chest pain**. Please keep in mind that my home town's altitude is 5280' above sea level. I'll be 75 next October.*

Thought you'd be interested to read about this.

Yours truly,   *F.W.*

Dear Dr. Rath:

Thank you for coming to share your knowledge and wisdom with us on your recent visit to the Northwest. My family and I are so grateful to you for your work and accomplishment preventing heart disease. We were introduced to your cardiovascular health program in February, and my husband and I are feeling better than we have felt in years. My husband had triple bypass surgery seven years ago and now we are confident that he won't have to repeat that procedure again.

*Our sister-in-law was diagnosed with congestive heart failure and told by her physician to go home and get her affairs in order, sell her home and prepare to move into a nursing home because she was only going to get worse and wouldn't be able to care for herself. **Her chest was full of fluids, she had to sleep sitting up, she was too weak to walk and her legs were swelling.***

(continued)

She started your cardiovascular health program late in February, and **_in three weeks she was feeling well enough to go out for dinner,_** *get her hair done and put her house on the market. She has since moved into a nice retirement home and* **_she goes everywhere the bus goes._**

She is so grateful, she has been given her life back and never wants to be without your cardiovascular health program.

She is 80 years old!

Sincerely,   *R.A.*

Dear Dr. Rath:

*I am a 46 year old female. Six years ago I had a severe reaction to a prescription medication. The ultimate result of that is that I had severe **congestive heart failure**. When I did not respond as rapidly as expected to digitalis and other medications, further tests showed more damage. Either due to the reactions or a previous bout with streptococcal bacteria, I was diagnosed as having valvular regurgitation of the mitral, tricuspid and pulmonary valves, as well as mitral valve prolapse. **My clinical symptoms were extreme fatigue, shortness of breath, edema, tachycardia and pulmonary edema.***

My cardiologist once remarked that I certainly did not need to have coronary artery disease, so I started on a fiber product and lowered my cholesterol from 215 to 148. I have responded fairly well to the medical regimen of my cardiologist. I have five teenagers at home when all this began. It was my best hope that I would be around and functioning to see all of them grow.

(continued)

When I first learned about your cardiovascular health program I was so overcome with emotion that I had to leave the room. It was too much to dream that there might be something that would allow one to live a full life and not just "exist."

__Since following your program I am now taking only a betablocker for medication. All others have been stopped__. My symptoms are now occasional fatigue that is easily fixed by a nap. I do not have severe shortness of breath, I can carry on a conversation without sounding out of breath. I am able to use the Nordic Track on a daily basis. __There is no edema, tachycardia, pulmonary congestion, etc.__

My youngest child just graduated from high school and is off to college soon. I own two companies, am in the process of writing a book, and can now look forward to many other adventures. Your cardiovascular health program has given me an entirely new look on the future, where at one time I did not feel that there would be a future.

Sincerely,   *J.T.*

Dear Dr. Rath:

I started your cardiovascular health program the same week I read your book titled "Why Animals Don't Get Heart Attacks, But Humans do." Unlike many things in this world, your presentations are so basic and simple that everyone can understand the principles involved.

My hope is that everyone in this country and the world will receive your message and have the same good results that I do.

I have eliminated my diuretic medications completely and cut my blood pressure medication in half since I started following your program. *I'm now reading 120 over 78 at age 69 and I feel great.*

My doctor was surprised and pleased and told me by all means to continue the preventative health care path that started with your program. *This program is unique and your patent on the technology to reverse heart disease without surgery is, as you say, like patenting nature — and it works.*

(continued)

Thank you so much for your work and for sharing your research with so many people. The world will be a happier place because of you.

Sincerely,   *B.B.*

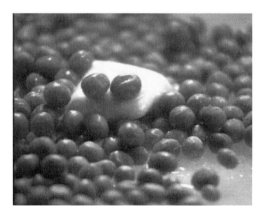

Peas are a good source of complex carbohydrates and proteins. Green peas have fair amounts of vitamin C, B-vitamins, also iron, potassium, and calcium

Dear Dr. Rath:

I am a 36 year old, Caucasian female. Since my late 20's I have experienced arrhythmia, shortness of breath periods. I also had begun to have edema in my ankles. My heart rate was usually between 88 and 98. My blood pressure averaged 140/86. Being a nurse, I knew to discontinue salt and caffeine. Upon doing so, the symptoms improved for a while. The past few years, however, I was beginning to require medication and was about to get further medical attention to my cardiac changes when I was introduced to your cardiovascular health program last February.

Now, four months later, I no longer require medication for the edema, nor do I have any arrhythmia, shortness of breath, or palpitations. *I have always continued my*

(continued)

aerobic exercise, which I was beginning to have difficulty in sustaining. However, my stamina has improved tremendously over these past few months. My heart rate now averages 78 and my blood pressure was 112/60 last week.

Thank you!

Sincerely and in Good Health,   *V.G.*

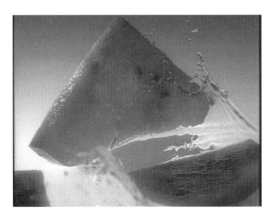

Watermelons are almost entirely composed of water and nutrients. They are high in beta carotene, vitamin C, potassium and magnesium.

Dear Dr. Rath:

For three months now I have been taking double the amounts of nutritional supplements recommended in your cardiovascular health program.

*I just returned from my usual 4-mile walk at a brisk pace, up two small hills (60' and 40' respectfully) and around the neighborhood **with no discomfort at all. For the first time absolutely free of distress.** This feels like a miracle!*

Best wishes,   *J.H.*

Dear Dr. Rath:

I knew about L-carnitine and coenzyme Q10 and was taking them, but I did not know as yet about L-proline or L-lysine or some of the other ingredients in your cardiovascular health program. I had devised a rather elaborate program for myself which involved a lot of tiring shopping from drug store to health food store, in order to buy what I thought I needed. Your cardiovascular health program pulled it all together for me. When I heard of it I said "how wonderful," a doctor who actually cares about health.

__The most important thing I have noticed since following your program is: no more shortness of breath__

Keep up the good work, Dr. Rath, and thank you for helping me extend and enrich my life.

Sincerely,   *W.S.*

Dear Dr. Rath:

*I am happy to report that your cardiovascular health program has improved my life. **Now I can climb the stairs readily and without shortness of breath**.*

I can also resume hiking for 3-4 miles a day without feeling tired and exhausted. I do have an energetic outlook towards life and sure it's due to your cardiovascular health program.

Thank you very much for all the research you have done and you are continuing to do for people with circulatory problems.

Sincerely,   *A.G.*

Cellular Medicine -

Breakthrough for Patients with High Blood Pressure

The Facts About High Blood Pressure

- **More than fifty million Americans** currently suffer from high blood pressure conditions. Among all health conditions, this is the single largest epidemic in America. Worldwide hundreds of millions of people suffer from high blood pressure conditions. The epidemic spread of this disease is largely due to the fact that until now the causes for high blood pressure have been insufficiently or not at all understood.

- **Conventional Medicine** is largely confined to treating the *symptoms* of this disease. Betablockers, diuretics and other high blood pressure medication target the symptoms of high blood pressure, not its underlying cause.

- **Cellular Medicine provides a breakthrough in our understanding of the causes of high blood pressure.** High blood pressure conditions are frequently caused or aggravated by a deficiency in vitamins and other essential nutrients in millions of vascular wall cells. Among other functions, these cells are responsible for the production of 'relaxing factors' which decrease vascular wall tension and keep the blood pressure in a normal range. Deficiencies of vitamins and other essential nutrients impair the function of the vascular wall cells, frequently resulting in spasms and thickening of the blood vessel walls and in elevated blood pressure.

- **Scientific research and clinical studies** have already documented the particular value of vitamin C, magnesium, coenzyme Q-10, arginine and other essential nutrients in helping to normalize high blood pressure conditions.

- **America's Most Successful Cardiovascular Health Program** comprises selected essential nutrients which are needed for optimum function of cells, including millions of vascular wall cells. The following pages document health improvements from patients with high blood pressure disease who have greatly benefited from this program.

- **My recommendations for patients with high blood pressure conditions**: Start immediately with this program and inform your doctor about it. Take the essential nutrients *in addition to* your regular medication. Do not stop your regular medication without consulting your doctor. Document your health improvements with this program.

112

High Blood Pressure

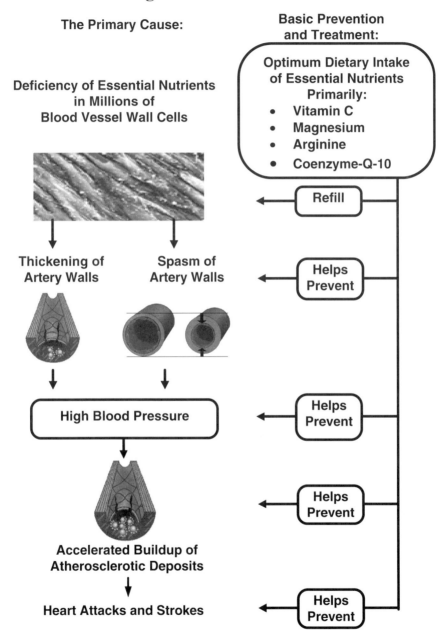

The Primary Cause:

Basic Prevention and Treatment:

Deficiency of Essential Nutrients in Millions of Blood Vessel Wall Cells

Optimum Dietary Intake of Essential Nutrients Primarily:
- Vitamin C
- Magnesium
- Arginine
- Coenzyme-Q-10

Refill

Thickening of Artery Walls

Spasm of Artery Walls

Helps Prevent

High Blood Pressure

Helps Prevent

Accelerated Buildup of Atherosclerotic Deposits

Helps Prevent

Heart Attacks and Strokes

Helps Prevent

Dear Dr. Rath:

About 8 weeks ago I was introduced to a fiber product for the reduction of my cholesterol, which had reached 260 in spite of efforts to get it down. After being on that product about 2 and a half weeks, I realized that my blood pressure was going up. **<u>I am on blood pressure medication for essential hypertension since my teen years</u>***. I supposed that it was due to the energy I was feeling from the fiber formula.*

Then I heard about your cardiovascular health program and that it had lowered blood pressure. I immediately started on your program. **<u>Within two weeks my blood pressure had gone from 145/150 over 90/96 to 130/82</u>*** - sometimes a bit higher if I am really busy! I noticed a lessening of a feeling of chest pressure also, and I could breathe deeper.*

Sincerely,   *S.S.*

Health improvement in 35 year old woman:

Elevated blood pressure readings for 4 months of around 150/112. Three different prescriptions by her physician would not reduce blood pressure readings. She also was having side effects from blood pressure medication. ***After starting your cardiovascular health program the blood pressure went to normal in 21 days and has remained normal for 3 months.***

Sincerely,   *J.L.*

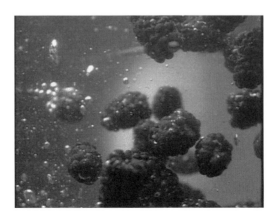

Both red and black raspberries are a good source of vitamin C, they are especially abundant in the minerals: calcium, magnesium and iron.

Dear Dr. Rath:

I started your cardiovascular health program the same week I read your book titled "Why Animals Don't Get Heart Attacks, But Humans Do." Unlike many things in this world, your presentations are so basic and simple that everyone can understand the principles involved.

My hope is that everyone in this country and the world will receive your message and have the same good results that I do.

__I have eliminated my diuretic medications completely and cut my blood pressure medication in half since I started following your program.__ I'm now reading 120 over 78 at age 69 and I feel great.

__My doctor was surprised and pleased and told me by all means to continue the preventative health care path that I started with your program.__ This program is unique and your patent on the technology to reverse heart disease without surgery is, as you say, like patenting nature - and it works.

Thank you so much for your work and for sharing your research with so many people. The world will be a happier place because of you.

Sincerely,   *B.B..*

Dear Dr. Rath,

*I am a 52-year old male with a **high blood pressure problem that spans 25 years**. I've been through six different physicians and I've lost count of the different blood pressure medications that have been prescribed for me.*

The best that any doctor was able to reduce my blood pressure to was an average of 135/95 for the last five or six years with a combination of prescription medication. When I first became aware of my high blood pressure, I was 27 years old and it was in the range of 165/125. Sound like a problem about to happen? I'm not overweight (never have been, ranging from 175 to 191 at 6'2") and I'm fairly active.

I began following your cardiovascular health program last December. My cholesterol prior to your program was 246. A month after starting your program my cholesterol was 288. I couldn't get an answer to the 288 from anyone at the time, but I had enough other positives (blood pressure reduction, more energy, arthritic problem vanished) that I

(continued)

didn't give up on either product and, after another month, the cholesterol went to 211. Thank you for the explanation. Now I won't be ashamed to talk about the 288

My blood pressure dropped to an average of 124/82 by the first week of January, along with a greater feeling of energy and well-being. That occurred despite no change in diet or lifestyle. ***My doctor reduced one of my blood pressure medications by half and my blood pressure still dropped over the next few months to an average of 122/80.***

The third week of May last year, it dropped to 120/64. So far, that level seems to be the start of a trend, so I'll have to visit my doctor again for a further reduction in medication. Along with the blood pressure reduction has come a reduction in a long-standing heavy perspiration problem I've had.

My best judgment tells me that this little embarrassing problem is 10% of what it has been for the last twenty-five years. I'm now comfortable wearing something other than white shirts!

(continued)

I am now absolutely convinced that your cardiovascular health program did really help to lower my blood pressure and all I can say is big 'Thank You'.

Sincerely,   *L.M.*

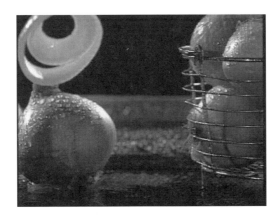

Onions are high in nutrients such as proteins, calcium, iron, folic acid, vitamin C, E, and A. They are also a source of selenium and zinc.

Dear Dr. Rath,

I have been following your cardiovascular health program for seven months. The calves of my legs were very sore.

*After 3 months the soreness is gone and I can push or even hit them with a fist and they do not hurt any more. Also, more importantly, **I am no longer on blood pressure medication.***

After 6 months on your program I am in the 130s over the 70s.

Thank you, Dr. Rath,

M.W.

Health improvement in 53 year old man:

His blood pressure was being controlled by blood pressure medication. He had been taking blood pressure medication of various types for 10 years.

After 4 months on your cardiovascular health program, this patient went off blood pressure medication, *while his blood pressure was checked every two weeks. His blood pressure has now been normal for 6 weeks, only with your cardiovascular health program.*

He had noticed some angina prior to this program, and those symptoms have also been eliminated.

Sincerely,   *J.L.*

Dear Dr. Rath,

I have been following your cardiovascular health program for five months.

In the meantime my doctor reduced my blood pressure medication by half *so I can honestly say I'm now taking half the medication than five months ago.*

I am maintaining blood pressure average of 120/78. Thrilled? You'd better believe it!

Next goal: no medication at all.

Thank you again.

Sincerely, *L.M.*

Cellular Medicine -

Breakthrough for Diabetic Patients

The Facts About Adult Diabetes

- **Several million Americans** have currently been diagnosed with Diabetes. Diabetic disorders have a genetic background and are divided into juvenile and adult types. Juvenile diabetes is generally caused by an insufficient production of insulin in the body and insulin injections have become a live-saving therapy for these patients. The great majority of diabetic patients, however, develop this disease as adults. Thus far, the causes which unmask the genetic disorder in adults and which trigger the onset of adult diabetes have been insufficiently understood.

- **Conventional Medicine** is largely confined to treating the *symptoms* of adult diabetes, e.g. by lowering elevated blood levels of sugar. However, cardiovascular diseases and other diabetic complications occur even in those patients with controlled blood sugar levels. This fact shows that the conventional understanding of this disease is still incomplete.

- **Cellular Medicine provides a breakthrough in our understanding of the causes of irregular heartbeat**. Adult onset diabetes is frequently caused or aggravated by a deficiency of certain vitamins and other essential nutrients in millions of cells in pancreas, liver, vascular wall, and in other organs. On the basis of an inherited diabetic disorder, deficiencies of vitamins and other essential nutrients can trigger a diabetic metabolism and the onset of adult diabetes.

- **Scientific research and clinical studies** have already documented the particular value of vitamin C, vitamin E, certain B-vitamins, chromium and other essential nutrients in helping to normalize a diabetic metabolism and to prevent cardiovascular diseases.

- **America's Most Successful Cardiovascular Health Program** comprises selected essential nutrients which are needed for optimum function of cells, including millions of cells in the pancreas, the liver and the vascular wall. The following pages document health improvements from diabetic patients who have greatly benefited from this program.

- **My recommendations for diabetic patients**: Start immediately with this program and inform your doctor about it. Take the essential nutrients *in addition to* your diabetes medication and take them regularly. Do not stop your prescription medication without consulting your doctor. Document your health improvements with this natural program.

124

Cardiovascular Complications in Diabetes (Adult Form)

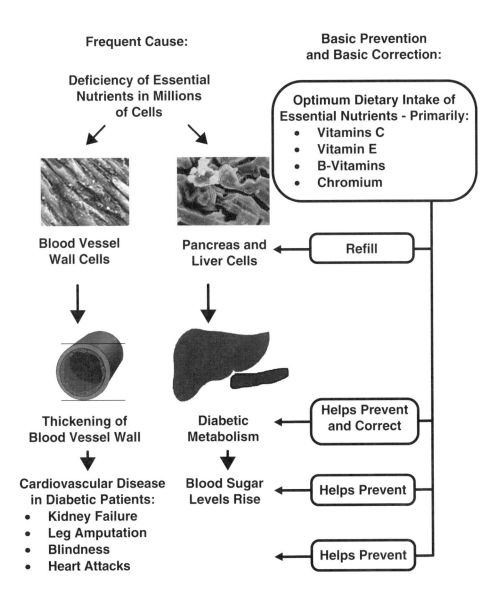

Frequent Cause:

Basic Prevention and Basic Correction:

Deficiency of Essential Nutrients in Millions of Cells

Optimum Dietary Intake of Essential Nutrients - Primarily:
- Vitamins C
- Vitamin E
- B-Vitamins
- Chromium

Blood Vessel Wall Cells

Pancreas and Liver Cells ← Refill

Thickening of Blood Vessel Wall

Diabetic Metabolism ← Helps Prevent and Correct

Cardiovascular Disease in Diabetic Patients:
- Kidney Failure
- Leg Amputation
- Blindness
- Heart Attacks

Blood Sugar Levels Rise ← Helps Prevent

← Helps Prevent

Dear Dr. Rath,

I started following your cardiovascular health program three months ago. I'm 29 years old and was recently diagnosed with **_Type II Diabetes._**

Since following your program on a regular basis, I have found my blood glucose level to remain around 100, even when under stress which previously raised my blood glucose level.

Your cardiovascular health program and 1-2 extra grams of vitamin C have relieved the primary negative symptoms that I have experienced such as weakness from low blood sugar levels, pain in the right side from high blood sugar, and painful urination from the higher blood sugar levels.

I have found only positive results from your program.

Sincerely,   *A.M.*

Dear Dr. Rath,

*I would like to share my story with you. This is in hope that the information will help other diabetics with similar conditions. More importantly, **I am hopeful this information will keep other diabetics from ever having to experience the frustration and debilitating pain involved with peripheral neuropathy**, as I have.*

My husband and I own and operate a catering business. In our business, I spend much time on my feet because it is a demanding, high stress, long hours job. For many years I have been suffering from diabetes and diabetic neuropathy. My toes were turning dark blue and purple, and I did not have any feeling in them. The prognosis was very grim; if my condition did not get any better I could lose my toes, if not my feet.

*I was looking for a treatment that would help this condition. Then I learned about your cardiovascular health program. **After about a week of following your program, to my delight, my toes became a bright maroon color instead of blue and purple**, and much to*

(continued)

my amazement hair was beginning to grow again on my legs. Like most women the hair on my legs didn't excite me from a glamour standpoint, but it did tell me that blood was reaching the hair follicles.

By the 2nd week my legs were not cramping as often or as badly but by the end of the 3rd week my feet and ankles were giving me excruciating pain. I mentioned what was happening to me to a friend who is a druggist. He grinned and happily told me that he believed the nerves were regenerating. Wasn't that great? I've spoken to professionals who are knowledgeable in treating diabetics and they are encouraging me to hang in there and stick with your program.

The feeling, which has been absent for several years, is coming back in my feet. *I can feel the inside of my shoes again. I am now starting the 3rd month on your program. My feet and legs still are very painful, but it's a coming back to life feeling and I look forward to wearing pretty shoes and hose occasionally instead of white cotton socks and heavily padded walking shoes.*   (continued)

*__More important than the glamour aspect
is the fact that I know I almost lost my feet__, which would have been devastating to anyone.*

Your cardiovascular health program, coupled with my stationery bicycle and insulin adjustments, suggestions from my dietitian, are all elements in helping me fight the battle and winning.

Very sincerely yours,   *M.J.*

Dear Dr. Rath,

In order to place my judgment of your cardiovascular health program in the proper perspective, a bit of history is in order. I am a 55 year old male Caucasian, weighing 154 pounds. I lead a very sedentary lifestyle spending most of my time sitting behind a desk in front of a computer.

*About 20 years ago I was diagnosed a **type II (adult onset) Diabetic** and placed on oral medication and dietary restrictions to control my blood sugar level. These precautions seemed to work up to about a year ago when my blood sugar went to about 260 where it remains fairly steady, a fact that caused my physician (an endocrinologist) to change my medication and to drastically increase my dosage. He is currently seeing me on a monthly basis in an attempt to stabilize my condition. According to his diagnosis I must control my diet much better than I have been doing up to now, and I must lose about 20 pounds (easier said than done).*

*In February of 1986, **I underwent quintuple bypass surgery to remedy severe angina** and.*

(continued)

all the other symptoms of cardiovascular disease. The operation was performed in time to forestall a heart attack, and since the operation I have not experienced any symptoms such as pain, shortness of breath or irregular heartbeat.

*I have followed your cardiovascular health program religiously, every day as prescribed in your instructions for exactly 2 months, and **since approximately 2 weeks ago I noticed a dramatic increase in my energy level. I can accomplish much more in my daily work, I find myself eager to stay up late,** and recently I found myself out dancing late at night with my wife, just as I used to do about 20 years ago.*

Since nothing in my daily routine has changed except the advent of your program. I must conclude that this newly found "fountain of youth" is a direct result of your formulation.

In closing, I am grateful to your cardiovascular health program for the improvements shown thus far and, needless to say, I am looking forward with anticipation to more improvements, specially in my ability to walk.

Please feel free to use this letter, or any part thereof as a testimonial in your efforts.

Sincerely,   *N.M.*

- Thus far you have had an opportunity to read about the health improvement with my Cardiovascular Health Program in patients with some form of cardiovascular disease. It is important to understand that any natural health program that is able to help correct so many cardiovascular conditions is also able to help prevent these conditions in the first place.

- The Cardiovascular Health Program I developed is above all a *preventive program for everyone* who wants to optimize cardiovascular health naturally. The following pages document the letters from people who followed my program for preventive purposes.

- Some of the following letters report health improvements like 'freer breathing' or 'less heaviness in the chest'. I encourage everyone with such symptoms, in addition to starting this program, to consult with a doctor.

Cellular Medicine -

Breakthrough in
the Prevention
of Cardiovascular Diseases

Dear Dr. Rath,

I am 29 years old and do not have heart problems as far as I know. I am "big" into health and supplements so I know quite a bit about vitamins and what I want from them. Yours are impressive - I intend to continue using them and I commend you on your development.

I have noticed increased energy, increased stamina, improved mental attitude, and a sense of freer breathing in my chest area. *I have never been able to run for very long because I would run out of breath (even as a child). However, I never thought it was due to my heart.*

I still don't know why, but what I do know is that I can jog on my mini-trampoline for a longer period of time and with greater ease after taking your vitamins. Before every minute seemed like three. Now it's much easier.

Thank you again.

Sincerely,   *J.M.*

Dear Dr. Rath:

I just turned 55 years old and I started following your cardiovascular health program in February. In April, I suddenly realized that I had a strong desire to run again. I started doing some racing in our back yard with my grandchildren. It dawned on me that I wasn't that winded, and I felt so agile compared to how I had been feeling.

For a number of years, I would avoid hiking, especially uphill, because I would get so winded that I could hardly breathe. *It was a scary feeling.*

A week ago, I went hiking with a friend who had a knee replacement a year ago and wanted to see if she should still do some hiking. ***In less than 2 days we hiked a good ten miles***. *I feel that the credit goes to your cardiovascular health program, since I am not on any other product or medication. I have never liked taking traditional medicines. This program would be the answer to many problems that people face when it comes to their health. As I lose more weight, I'm sure*

(continued)

that my energy and stamina will be even better.

By the way, I had a physical the end of May and they gave me an EKG. They said everything was normal. I press on to a healthier life style.

Thanks, Dr. Rath, for your time in researching and developing a health program that has changed so many lives.

Sincerely,   *L.H.*

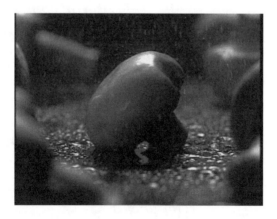

Many mushrooms are high in iron and selenium. Biotin, niacin, folic acid and pantothenic acid are also in good quantities in mushrooms.

Dear Dr. Rath,

I started your cardiovascular health program two months ago. What I have noticed is that I do have __more energy and stamina__ and

I am able to stay on a job longer than before. This is very encouraging.

Sincerely,   *M.L*

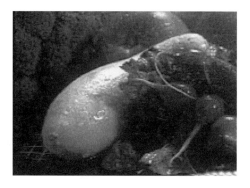

Squashes are rich in starch and fiber. Many are high in vitamin A (orange or yellow squash), vitamin C and potassium

Dear Dr. Rath,

*I have been following your cardiovascular health program for four months now. I am and have been a manager for nine years, dealing with stress and have smoked for 20 years. In addition, **my family has a history of heart disease** and high blood pressure.*

*Approximately three weeks after starting your cardiovascular health program **I noticed that I was no longer experiencing the 'heaviness' in my chest in the morning that I had previously experienced**. I credit this change to the benefits received from your program! I do not have medical proof to back up my testimonial, but do know I feel better and that's enough for me! Also, I'm pleased my father, who has had heart surgery and associated problems, choose to get on the program.*

Thank you for your continued dedication to improving America's health, Dr. Rath, I wish you continued success.

Sincerely,   *C.G.*

Dear Dr. Rath:

Although I do not have any apparent heart problems, I have had some breathing difficulty due to emphysema. My past nasty habit of smoking, and the resulting abuse, is apparently responsible for this condition.

Because I am a healthy 68-year-old, except for the emphysema, my breathlessness has been limited to hill climbing on my daily 3-mile walk and while doing heavy work, but has been cause for apprehension.

After the first month on your cardiovascular health program it became apparent that I was having less trouble with breathlessness, which appears to be continually improving.

I'm pleased, and I shall continue to follow this program.

Yours truly,   *I.J.*

The Facts About Cholesterol

Cholesterol has received much attention as an indicator of cardiovascular risk. Cholesterol levels are determined by three main factors: genetic disposition, dietary fat intake, and by the dietary supplementation of vitamins and other essential nutrients. Our new understanding of cardiovascular disease shows that cholesterol and other blood factors only become risk factors, when the artery walls are weakened by too little vitamin intake over many years.

We now also know that there is a close connection between the stability of the blood vessel wall and the production rate of cholesterol and other *repair* factors in the liver. A rise in cholesterol levels frequently reflects an additional need of the body to repair the vitamin deficient and instable blood vessel walls. Thus, if the vascular wall is weakened by vitamin deficiency, the need for overproduction of cholesterol in the liver increases and cholesterol levels in the blood rise.

In contrast, if the vascular wall is stabilized with optimum intake of vitamins and other essential nutrients, the liver produces fewer repair molecules and the levels of cholesterol in the blood decreases. Moreover, scientific research has shown that vitamin C decreases the production of cholesterol in the body and also accelerates its elimination through the liver. Cholesterol levels may be further lowered by combining these essential nutrients with fiber-rich nutrition or a fiber formula.

Most people who start my cardiovascular program report a decrease in cholesterol and other risk factors. In other people cholesterol levels remain constant for some time and then drop.

In some people, however cholesterol levels rise when they enter this cardiovascular program. Since vitamin supplementation decreases cholesterol production in the liver, the additional cholesterol measured in the blood must derive from deposits in the artery walls and in other tissues. This mechanism was first described by Dr. Constance Spittle in the medical journal *The Lancet* in 1972. After a few months on the vitamin program cholesterol levels generally drop below the initial value (see letters).

Cholesterol lowering alone, without stabilizing the vascular wall with vitamins and other essential nutrients, is an incomplete approach to cardiovascular health. The Cardiovascular Health Program documented in this book is the basis to achieve cardiovascular health naturally.

Dear Dr. Rath,

Heart disease is hereditary within my family and my father had his first heart attack in his early thirties.

*I had my cholesterol checked at age 19 only to find out that **I had a cholesterol level of 392**. My physician did not want to place me on medication at that time, so I just watched my diet and increased my exercise. Well, as time passed, my cholesterol remained elevated and my physician felt medication was necessary. I refused to begin medication and continued with diet and exercise.*

*At age 26 I had my cholesterol tested before I began your program, and my lab test showed a reading of 384. I immediately **began following your program, including a fiber product, and my level dropped 120 points within a 6-10 week period. Over a four month period, my LDL went from 308 down to 205.***

Now there is a program which I personally follow and continue to have positive results with. I recommend it to my family and friends.

Sincerely,   *C.C.*

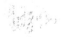

Dear Dr. Rath,

I had started taking a fiber product in February of 1994. My cholesterol continued to climb from 280 to over 320 until May of 1994, when I began to follow your cardiovascular health program.

My cholesterol has dropped to 180, my ratio of HDL to LDL is normal as is my triglyceride level. Most important, however, my lipoprotein(a) dropped from 15 to 1! *I will continue your program forever.*

Thank you, Dr. Rath, for your work with natural products as a means to decreasing the risk of heart disease.

With much gratitude,   *M.R.*

Dear Dr. Rath,

I am 45 years old and since December last year I have been on your cardiovascular health program and I also take a fiber product.

<u>Last April my cholesterol level was 259. This April, after only 4 months on this program, my cholesterol dropped to 175!</u>

Dr. Rath, I truly want to thank you for helping me to be healthier and able to live a much fuller life. I am looking forward to turning 45 because I am in such excellent physical condition.

We all wish you continued success in your research and development to help all of us be healthier human beings.

Sincerely,   *M.W.*

Dear Dr. Rath,

I began taking a fiber formula two years ago, in September. My total cholesterol was around **177** at that time. Within 90 days, I lost 20 lbs. and my total cholesterol level dropped to **154**.

In November last year I started with your Cardiovascular Health Program. An insurance physical that was done in February this year showed a total cholesterol level of **191**, triglycerides 244. LDL/HDL ratio of 4.09. CHOL/HDL ratio of 6.8, all which were elevated. Again, note that this was February.

A cholesterol screening was done in March and again in June. Both showed a total cholesterol level of **134**. A lipid profile that was done in July showed total cholesterol level 135, triglycerides 180. LDL/HDL ratio of 1.47, and **CHOL/HDL ratio down to 3.16 from 6.8**.

Your Cardiovascular Health Program is working!

Sincerely,   L.M.

Dear Dr. Rath,

I have been on your cardiovascular health program since April. Today, I received the results of my follow-up blood test and, in just under sixty days, my cholesterol has dropped as follows:

	Cholesterol	*Triglycerides*
Before April	*242*	*3 times normal*
June	*169*	*106*

Thank you so much for your discovery. I have added vitamin C along with antioxidants and it worked out just fine.

Several of my friends are now on your program and were astounded when I informed them of the outcome within 60 days.

Wishing you continued success in all your endeavors.

Sincerely,   *L.K.*

Other Encouraging Letters

Dear Dr. Rath:

*My father, who is 84, has **<u>Alzheimer's Disease</u>**. About two months ago his care givers attended an Alzheimer's seminar at a nursing home there. The seminar reported that some patients had been put on a vitamin supplement program which had resulted in improved memory for several patients. We compared ingredients and decided that your cardiovascular health program offered more than what was used at the nursing home.*

***<u>My father has been on this program for two months and we cannot believe the improvement. His short term memory is improving and we can carry on conversations with him again. He is even showing some problem solving capabilities again</u>**. I know these improvements are not measurable from a "pure scientific perspective" but to us it's a blessing to see improvement rather than just deterioration from this terrible disease.*

On behalf o my father and our family, thank you for your cardiovascular health program.

Yours truly,   *D.C.*

Dr. Rath,

I have been so excited to learn more and more about your research. To say that it's compelling is an understatement.

I've been a Registered Nurse for 21 years, certified in critical care and emergency nursing. My real passion has been cardiology and cardiac rehabilitation in recent years.

I'm excited for my patients because your work is going to give them hope. Most of them are very compliant with diet and exercise, but continue to have hypercholesterolemia, hyperglycemia, etc.

Your cardiovascular health program will change their lives.

Sincerely,   T.E., RN

Dear Dr. Rath:

Your most interesting, informative publications in the Journal of Orthomolecular Medicine during 1991 till 1993, introduced the interested in the most promising therapeutic world for cardiovascular diseases.

The results of your scientific approach in your vitamin C research programs should be considered as an award-winning completion of the vitamin C odyssey, started by James Lind and followed by Irwin Stone, Linus Pauling and Emanuel Cheraskin.

Sincerely   *A.H., M.D., Ph.D.*

America's Most Successful Cardiovascular Health Program

-

Compared to Other Approaches

Biological Targets for Prevention of Cardiovascular Disease
- Conventional Medicine -

America's Most Successful Cardiovascular Health Program stands any comparison with other preventive cardiovascular approaches. Preventive approaches by conventional medicine focus on cholesterol-lowering, reduction of other risk factors, and on life style changes. None of these approaches targets the decisive biological problem - the instability of the vascular walls which triggers atherosclerotic deposits.

Cardiovascular prevention programs based on lifestyle changes *alone* are limited by the fact that they lack key targets of cardiovascular health such as optimum antioxidant protection, optimum vascular stability and repair, as well as optimum resupplementation of cell fuels.

**Biological Targets
of Conventional Medicine
A. Inside the Artery Wall**
- ?
- ?
- ?
- ?
- ?
- ?
- ?

B. In the Blood Circulation
- **Lowering of Cholesterol**
- ?
- ?

Healthy Lifestyle
- **Healthy Diet**
- **Regular Physical Activity**
- **Time to Relax**
- **Stop Smoking**

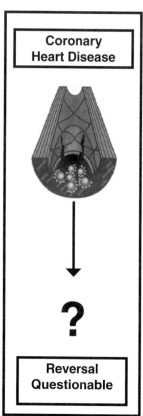

Coronary
Heart Disease

?

Reversal
Questionable

Biological Targets for Prevention of Cardiovascular Disease
- Cellular Medicine -

In contrast, the vitamins and other essential nutrients in my cardiovascular health program have defined biological targets. No other preventive health program currently available anywhere targets the main problem, the atherosclerotic deposits, in such a direct and comprehensive way: Vascular wall stability is optimized, vascular healing processes are induced, antioxidant and "teflon" protection is provided. The most important biological targets of this natural cardiovascular health program are summarized below.

It is the scientific basis of this natural program that will make this cardiovascular health program a basic health care option for thousands of doctors and other health care professionals across America.

**Biological Targets
of Cellular Medicine**

A. Inside the Artery Wall
- **Stability of Artery Walls**
- **Repair Processes**
- **Reversal of Deposits**
- **'Teflon'- Protection**
- **Antioxidant Protection**
- **Bioenergy for Wall Cells**
- **Relaxation of Artery Wall**

B. In the Blood Circulation
- **Lowering of Risk Factors**
- **Optimum Blood Viscosity**
- **Optimum Blood Cell Function**

Healthy Lifestyle
- **Healthy Diet**
- **Regular Physical Activity**
- **Time to Relax**
- **Stop Smoking**

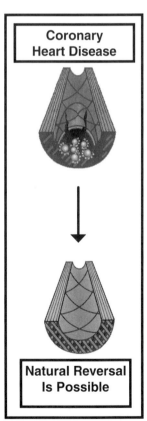

**Coronary
Heart Disease**

**Natural Reversal
Is Possible**

America's Most Successful Cardiovascular Health Program Compared to Other Programs
Biological Versatility

This figure illustrates the superior biological versatility of America's Most Successful Cardiovascular Health Program. This program provides the essential nutrients and cell fuels for millions of cardiovascular cells. This approach allows for prevention and correction of impaired cellular function in different compartments of the cardiovascular system *at the same time.*

Conventional therapy is frequently limited to the treatment of one cardiovascular symptom at a time. Since most heart disease patients have many cardiovascular problems they require several medications at the same time.

Note: This figure illustrates a biological principle. It does not mean that you can stop or substitute your prescription medication. **Always consult with your doctor about changing your medication.**

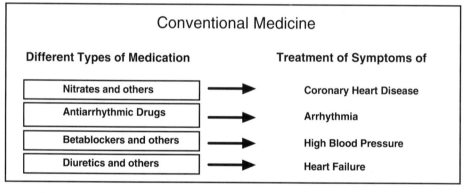

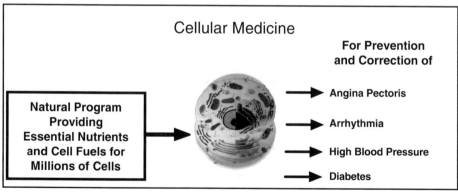

America's Most Successful Cardiovascular Health Program Compared to Other Programs
Safety

One of the greatest advantages of America's Most Successful Cardiovascular Health Program is that it is safe, and undesired side effects are essentially unknown. This is not surprising, since all the ingredients of this program are produced by Nature itself. For additional information on the safety of vitamins I recommend a recent review article in the Annals of the New York Academy of Sciences by Dr. A. Bendich.

In the figure below I have compared this natural program with preventive cardiovascular approaches offered by conventional medicine which are currently used by millions of Americans. The potential side effects are listed as well as the references where these potential side effects can be reviewed by everyone.

Conventional Medicine		
Preventive Approach	**Potential Side Effects**	**References**
Cholesterol Lowering Drugs (Statins)	Liver Damage, Myopathy	Physician's Desk Reference (PDR)
Cholesterol Lowering Drugs (Fibrates)	Liver Damage, Gastrointestinal Reactions	PDR
Aspirin	Ulcers, Stroke, Degrades Collagen	PDR Brooks (See Ref.)

Cellular Medicine		
Preventive Approach	**Potential Side Effects**	
Natural Cardiovascular Health Program	None	Bendich (See Ref.)

Vitamins and other essential nutrients have additional beneficial effects which patients on "blood thinning" medication and diabetic patients should know about: they help keep the blood at optimum viscosity and they help to normalize diabetic conditions. Inform your doctor. It is likely that *your doctor* can decrease your prescription medication. Do not change any medication on your own.

Milestones of Cellular Medicine

1859 Rudolf Virchow introduces "Cellular Pathology" - the scientific concept that diseases originate from malfunctioning cells. Cellular Pathology becomes one of the foundations of modern medicine. While the most frequent *cause* of diseases is now correctly identified - vitamins and essential nutrients remain to be discovered as the most frequent *remedy* of cellular malfunction and disease.

1920s-1940s The structure of most vitamins and other essential nutrients is solved. Many functions for each vitamin and essential nutrient are discovered at the biochemical level. However, these biochemical discoveries are insufficiently or not at all transferred to medical practice. Consequently, throughout this century, millions of people were deprived of live-saving information about the health benefits of vitamins and other essential nutrients.

The main reason for this unfortunate development is an economic one. Vitamins are not patentable and throughout the 20th century there was little economic incentive to invest in research and clinical studies with essential nutrients. Thus the outstanding health benefits of essential nutrients neither entered the media nor the medical schools, nor the daily medical practice of generations of physicians.

1960s-1980s Irvin Stone, Linus Pauling, Emanuel Cheraskin and others promote the use of vitamins against cancer, the common cold and dental disorders. However, the scientific and clinical evidence remains scarce.

1987-1992 Breakthrough in the area of cardiovascular disease and essential nutrients. Dr. Rath writes two scientific papers "Solution to the Puzzle of Human Cardiovascular Disease" and "A Unified Theory of Cardiovascular Disease" declaring for the first time that cardiovascular disease can be controlled by an optimum intake of vitamins and essential nutrients. Linus Pauling accepts invitation as co-author.

An increasing number of supportive clinical studies on the cardiovascular benefits of vitamins has become available.

1992 Health Now is founded as a research and development firm in nutritional medicine. The first formulas of vitamins and essential nutrients for optimizing cardiovascular health become available.

1993 Dr. Rath's book "Eradicating Heart Disease" is published. This book helps thousands of readers to better understand their body and introduces them to an effective "self-help" program to optimize cardiovascular health with essential nutrients. Most leading medical schools follow with their own "self-help" books for cardiovascular health. Even the American Heart Association now publishes a "self-help" health book. A truly healthy development for millions of Americans who have been disenfranchised from participating in their own body and health care for too long.

1994 With overwhelming public support the US Congress passes laws that ban efforts by the FDA to make many essential nutrients prescription items. Moreover, these laws now explicitly allow dissemination of scientific information about the health benefits of vitamins and other essential nutrients.

1994 Health Now develops a cardiovascular program specifically targeted to optimize cellular functioning. New marketing channels make this program accessible to over 20,000 Americans and establish America's Most Successful Cardiovascular Health Program.

1995 The scientific concept of Cellular Medicine is introduced in the June issue of Health Now's Newsletter. Thus the circle that started with Rudolf Virchow's pioneering work on Cellular Pathology is successfully closed and the age of Cellular Medicine is inaugurated.

The perspectives of Cellular Medicine are truly mind-boggling: The cellular architecture and the functioning of the human body will hardly change over the next millennia. Thus, Cellular Medicine and the scientific basis of America's Most Successful Cardiovascular Health Program will become an important foundation of Medicine for future generations.

Acknowledgments

I would like to thank all those who have contributed to this book in many ways. First and foremost to all those who sent their testimonial letters to me. Without You, this book would not exist.

I would like to acknowledge my colleagues at Health Now; Jeff Kamradt for his dedicated help in composing this book, Dr. Alexandra Niedzwiecki for critical review of the manuscript and Martha Best for outstanding secretarial help.

Special thanks go to Damon DeSantis and Armend Szmulewitz and to the distributors of Rexall Showcase International for their valuable contribution to this important process.

I also appreciate the help and courtesy of Al Fabrizio and Camera Graphics with the printing of this book.

I would also like to acknowledge the continued support from Dr. Roger Barth and Bernard Murphy for our efforts.

Selected References

The following list comprises selected publications about medical research and clinical studies documenting the health benefits of vitamins and other essential nutrients recommended in this book. This is only a selection of articles and further references can be found in my book *"Eradicating Heart Disease"*.

Cellular Medicine

Rath M. Why animals don't get heart attacks - but people do. 1994, Health Now, San Francisco.

Rath M. The new era of cellular medicine. Health Now Newsletter 1995, 5: 1-6, Health Now, San Francisco.

Cardiovascular Disease

Rath M. Reducing the risk of cardiovascular disease with nutritional supplements. Journal of Orthomolecular Medicine 1992; 7: 153-162.

Rath M. and Pauling L. Solution to the puzzle of human cardiovascular disease. Journal of Orthomolecular Medicine 1991, 6: 125-134.

Enstrom J.E.. Vitamin C intake and mortality among a sample of the United States population: New results. In New Strategies in Prevention and Therapy. K. Schmidt ed., Hippokrates Verlag Stuttgart 1994: 229-241.

Knekt P. et al. Antioxidant vitamin intake and coronary mortality in a longitudinal population study. American Journal of Epidemiology 1994, 1390: 1180-1189.

Stampfer M.J. et al. Vitamin E consumption and the risk of coronary disease in women. New England Journal of Medicine 1993, 328: 1444-1449.

Hodis H.N. et al. Serial angiographic evidence that antioxidant vitamin intake reduces progression of coronary artery atherosclerosis. Journal of the American Medical Association 1995, 273: 12849-1854.

Arrhythmia

Iseri L.T. Magnesium: nature's physiologic calcium blocker. American Heart Journal 1984, 108: 188-193.

Rizzon P. et al. High dose of L-carnitine in acute myocardial infarction: metabolic and antiarrhythmic effects. European Heart Journal 1989, 10: 502-508.

Gullestadt L. et al. The effect of magnesium versus verapamil on supraventricular arrhythmias. Clinical Cardiology 1993, 16: 429-434.

Heart Failure

Ghidini O. et al. Evaluation of the therapeutic efficacy of L-carnitine in congestive heart failure. International Journal of Clinical Pharmacology, Therapy and Toxicology 1988, 26: 217-220.

Folkers K and Yamamura Y (eds.). Biomedical and clinical aspects of coenzyme Q10. Volume 1-5, 1976-1986, Elsevier Science Publishers New York.

Wester P.O. et al. Intracellular electrolytes in cardiac failure. Acta Med. Scand. 1986, 707: 33-36.

High Blood Pressure

Mc Carron D.A. et al. Blood pressure and nutrient intake in the United States. Science 1984, 224: 1392-1398.

Jacques P.F. Effects of Vitamin C on high density lipoprotein, cholesterol and blood pressure. Journal of the American College of Nutrition 1993, 11: 139-144.

Langsjoen P.H. Isolated diastolic dysfunction of the myocardium and its response to CoQ10 treatment. Clinical Investigation 1993, 71: S140-S144.

Tarry W.C. L-Arginine improves endothelium-dependent vasorelaxation and reduces intimal hyperplasia after balloon angioplasty. Arteriosclerosis and Thrombosis 1994, 14: 938-943.

Diabetes

Pfleger R. and Scholl F. Diabetes and Vitamin C. Wiener Archiv fuer Innere Medizin 1937, 31: 219-230.

Mann G.V. et al. The membrane transport of ascorbic acid. Second Conference on Vitamin C Annals of the New York Academy of Sciences 1975: 243-252.

Liu V.J. Chromium and insulin in young subjects with normal glucose tolerance. American Journal of Clinical Nutrition 1982, 25: 661-667.

Kapeghian JC and Verlangieri J. The effects of glucose on ascorbic acid uptake in heart endothelial cells: possible pathogenesis of diabetic angiopathies. Life Sciences 1984, 34: 577-584.

Kodama M. et al. Diabetes Mellitus is controlled by vitamin C treatment. In Vivo 1993, 7: 535-542.

Cunningham J. et al. Vitamin C: an aldose reductase inhibitor that normalizes erythrocyte sorbitol in insulin-dependent diabetes mellitus. Journal of the American College of Nutrition 1994, 13: 344-350.

Cholesterol

Ginter E. Cholesterol: Vitamin C controls its transformation into bile acids. Science 1973, 179: 702.

Spittle C. Atherosclerosis and vitamin C. Lancet 1971,II: 1280-1281.

Aulinskas T.H. et al. Ascorbate increases the number of low density lipoprotein receptors in cultured arterial smooth muscle cells. Atherosclerosis 1983, 47: 159-171.

Harwood H.J. et al. Inhibition of human leucocyte 3-hydroxy-3-methylglutaryl coenzyme A reductase activity by ascorbic acid. An effect mediated by the free radical monohydroascorbate. Journal of Biological Chemistry 1986, 261: 7127-7135.

Hemilae H. Vitamin C and plasma cholesterol. In: Critical Reviews in Food Science and Nutrition 1992, 32 (1): 33-57. CRC Press. Boca Raton, FL.

Safety of Vitamins

Bendich A. In: Beyond Deficiency - New views on the function and health effects of vitamins. Annals of the New York Academy of Sciences 1992, 669: 300-312.

Side Effects of Drugs

Physician's Desk Reference Edition 1995, Medical Economics, Montvale NJ.

Brooks P.M. et al. Non-steroidal anti-inflammatory drugs and osteoarthritis - help or hindrance. Journal of Rheumatology 1982, 9: 3-5.